THE SUNDAY TIMES
SELF-HELP DIRECTORY

THE SUNDAY TIMES SELF-HELP DIRECTORY

Edited by

Judith Chisholm and Oliver Gillie

Foreword by

Jack Ashley C.H., M.P.

The research for this book was undertaken by Judith Chisholm and the bibliography was compiled by Nancy Bolton.

First published in Great Britain in 1975 by Times Newspapers Limited, New Printing House Square, London WC1X 8EZ

ISBN 7230 0142 1

Printed and bound in Great Britain by The Anchor Press Limited and Wm Brendon & Son Limited, both of Tiptree, Essex

Contents

Foreword

The sense of isolation created by social or medical problems often makes a difficult situation unbearable. Normal relationships with others are severed or impaired so that afflicted persons are denied help or encouragement when they need them most. As friendship is eroded and day-to-day contact reduced, people in desperate need are frequently left to their own resources.

The apparent indifference of society to human problems can be profoundly disturbing. People trying to grapple with a new disability or illness are sometimes dismayed to observe a world scurrying about its own business. Everyone is preoccupied with his own affairs and seems to have little time, and even less inclination, to help others. It is a sad and chastening new perspective on mankind.

Yet this picture is a fake. The general impression obscures latent kindness, genuine concern and, above all, practical help. Assistance is available, if people only know where to find it. The patchwork of State assistance and voluntary organisations has grown haphazardly throughout the years and has lain shrouded in a mist of vagueness – at least so far.

In this Directory the facts clearly emerge. There is a vast range of organisations catering for almost every problem. They vary in size, shape and method and some of them overlap. But they provide a valuable framework of self-help, encouragement and assistance for those in need. It is an overdue publication which will help to allay the anxieties and ease the burdens of many people.

JACK ASHLEY

Foreword

Introduction

This book is designed to help people to help themselves by providing contact with others who have similar problems and by providing access to sources of information. People with problems often become expert in practical means of coping with them. They have the advantage, over professionals, of firsthand experience. For this reason self-help organisations have earned an important place for themselves next to the professional help of doctors and social workers.

We have included organisations concerned with medical problems, disablement, social problems, problems of immigrants and problems of women and mothers. We hope this book will be especially useful to people with chronic illness or disability who have, in effect, been told that they must learn to live with their problem. We hope that through contact with others, and by reading about their problem, they will understand it better and be able to cope with it.

This directory only includes organisations which provide practical help or advice and appear to us to have a genuine point of view. The advice offered may sometimes be controversial, since there are often several quite different and equally valid approaches to the same illness or problem. In the end the person who obtains conflicting advice from professionals and others must judge the value of the advice for himself in the light of his own experience.

We have deliberately excluded organisations which are only interested in research or concerned only to act as pressure groups. We have also excluded religious organisations except when provision of practical help is their primary aim.

How to use the book

The book consists of four sections: (1) a directory of help which may be available from the State; (2) an alphabetical directory of organisations which aim to help people with problems; (3) a classified list of books which will provide information for those who want to know more about their problem; (4) a comprehensive index which will guide readers to sources of information or self-help organisations relevant to their problem.

TO FIND OUT MORE ABOUT A PARTICULAR PROBLEM, TURN TO THE INDEX FIRST: IT WILL REFER YOU TO PAGES IN THE OTHER SECTIONS OF THE BOOK WHERE RELEVANT ORGANISATIONS, BOOKS AND SOURCES OF HELP ARE LISTED.

General information about voluntary organisations can also be obtained from:

England	National Council of Social Service 26 Bedford Square London WC1 01 636 4066
Scotland	Scottish Council for Social Service 18/19 Claremont Crescent Edinburgh EH7 4HX 031 556 3882
Wales	Council of Social Service for Wales 2 Cathedral Road Cardiff CF1 9XR 0222 21456
Northern Ireland	Northern Ireland Council for Social Service 2 Annandale Avenue Belfast BT7 3JH 0232 643886/645489

Please help us

We plan to update this book each year. Please let us know of any changes of address or telephone number. We would also like to know of any new organisations which provide help, advice or counselling, and we would like to include others which we might have overlooked. Please send this information to Oliver Gillie, Medical Correspondent, the *Sunday Times*, 200 Gray's Inn Road, London WC1X 8EZ.

Acknowledgements

We would like to thank all the readers of the *Sunday Times* who responded to our call for help in preparing this directory and so made it possible. We would also like to thank the staff of the *Sunday Times* who have given us valuable information.

JUDITH CHISHOLM

OLIVER GILLIE

Section 1

How the State may help

1 Social Services

The Chronically Sick and Disabled Persons Act of 1970 has made it mandatory 'in the light of local resources' for local authorities to provide a wide variety of services for the old and handicapped. So it is wise, if in need, to consult first the Social Services Department of your local Council, listed in the telephone book under 'Health & Social Security, Dept. Of'. The address is also available from the Town Hall or local Library. Many of the organisations listed in this book also offer cash grants and practical aids to those living with a disablement.

The Disablement Income Group (D.I.G.), Queens House, 180/182a, Tottenham Court Road, London, W1P 0BD (01 636 1946/7) list in great detail the benfits and aids obtainable through the Social Services Departments of local Councils and some of them are given below. If you feel you could benefit from any of these aids get in touch with D.I.G. who will tell you whether you qualify and, if so, how to make a claim.

Adaptations to the Home
Ramps, rails, run-ins, etc., and major structural alterations to help disabled people.

Adult Training Centres
These offer simple training and social aids to severely subnormal adult people.

Aids and Equipment
For bath, toilet, dressing, walking, respiratory aids, hearing aids, kitchen gadgets, adjustable beds, pillows, dressing aids, make-up, specially adapted clothing.

Alarms
G.P.O. indicators, alarm systems to alert neighbours when in distress.

Appliances
Elastic hosiery, splints, calipers, footwear, surgical supports.

Attendance Allowance
A weekly allowance, non-contributory, non-means-tested and tax free, paid on medical grounds to severely disabled people (including children) who need a prescribed amount of care.

Badges
Special car badges are issued to disabled drivers with invalid tricycles or cars. Institutions with vehicles for use of disabled people are also eligible. These badges confer special parking privileges throughout the country except for five inner London areas where local disc schemes operate.

Bedding
A grant may be made to supplementary benefit claimants (also one for extra laundry cost).

Board and Lodging Allowance
An allowance paid to supplementary benefit claimants plus extra for personal expenses.

Child's Special Allowance
Paid for children of a divorced woman on the death of her former husband (if he was contributing to child's maintenance).

Clothing
A discretionary grant for essential clothing for a supplementary benefit claimant and dependants. Essential clothing for school children may be supplied by the local Education Department. Second-hand clothing is generally available through W.R.V.S. (address in this book), but a letter of recommendation is usually necessary.

Concessions
Certain disabled people are entitled to concessions on cinema tickets, launderettes, deck chairs, bowling greens, postage on books, etc.

Constant Attendance Allowance
Paid to severely disabled people who draw 100% disablement pensions under the Industrial Injury scheme.

Death Grant
A lump sum to meet funeral expenses paid to a dependant. In the case of a disabled person the grant may be claimed on insurance of a close relation.

Dental Charges
People and dependants drawing supplementary benefits or family income supplement or in receipt of a low income are exempt from dental charges.

Diet
An extra weekly discretionary allowance may be paid to supplementary benefit claimants.

Disposables
These can be supplied, as can incontinence pads, plastic bed sheets, special clothing, laundry services.

Domiciliary Care and Services
Home helps, home nursing, meals-on-wheels, physiotherapy, occupational therapy.

Earnings Related Supplement
Working widows and claimants earning over a specified sum in the previous year and eligible for sickness, unemployment or injury benefit, can claim extra supplement for six months.

Electrical Equipment
Special equipment is available to suit disabled people's needs.

Fares
People drawing supplementary benefit, family income supplement or with low income who must attend hospital or appliance centres for treatment may have their fares refunded. Discretionary help is also given with fares to visit sick relations in hospital or to send children of sick parents to relations. British Rail offer concessionary fares for visitors to long-term patients in hospital.

Furniture
Discretionary grants can sometimes be made to supplementary benefit claimants. Local Social Services Departments may have a stock of second-hand furniture.

Guardian's Allowance
Payable to guardians of orphaned children.

Heating Allowance
A weekly discretionary allowance for supplementary benefit claimants.

Holidays
These are sometimes organised by Social Services Departments, who may also subsidise a holiday.

Home Helps
No charge should be made to supplementary benefit claimants.

Home Nursing
A District Nurse will visit sick, disabled or elderly people, to bathe, etc., on recommendation of a doctor. There is no charge for this service.

House Decoration
A lump sum may be given further to supplementary benefit claimants.

Industrial Injuries
Paid to people injured at work or with certain illnesses arising through work. Entitlement is not dependent on number of National Insurance contributions.

Invalidity Benefit
A pension and allowance paid to sickness benefit claimants (if at least five years below retirement age) after 28 weeks and varying according to age at onset of incapacity. Increased children's allowances payable. Wife of an invalidity pensioner has a higher earning limit before husband's allowance for her is affected.

Library
Mobile Library Service. Books delivered to homes of housebound.

Long-Term Addition
A standard sum paid automatically to:
(a) Supplementary pensioners *unless* in hospital, boarders or people in Local Authority or similar accommodation.
(b) People who have received a supplementary allowance for two years previously without having to register for employment.

Luncheon Clubs
Run by various organisations and offering subsidised lunch.

Meals-on-Wheels
Hot meals delivered at subsidised rate to homes of eligible people at midday.

Milk
Liquid or dried milk free to handicapped children between 5 and 16 years who are not at school.

Night Sitters
Can be supplied for sick and infirm people.

Pensions for People over 80
A non-contributory pension for people not already drawing a National Insurance pension or who are drawing one only at a reduced rate.

Prescriptions
Ex-service disablement pensioners (if prescription relates to their pensioned disablement), people and their families on supplementary benefit or family income supplement are entitled to certificates of exemption from medical charges; refunds are also available on income grounds if prescription has already been paid for.

Removal
A lump sum may be paid towards the expense of this to supplementary benefit claimants.

Residential Homes
Can be provided by Social Services Department for old and disabled people. If they are unable to provide accommodation, they might help with fees of voluntary organisations like the Cheshire Homes.

Special Hardship Allowance
Paid to industrial injury pensioners if they are unable to return to former or similar job.

Supplementary Benefits
Although full-time work disqualifies claims for benefit, disabled self-employed people with greatly reduced earning power may apply for benefit.

Talking Book Service
May be available free to housebound disabled people.

Telephones
May be provided by Supplementary Benefit Commission (through Social Security Office) according to certain criteria, for example, the isolation of the disabled person in relation to degree of handicap. Special operating aids available.

Television
Rented sets for isolated, housebound, disabled people may be provided and help may also be given with licence fee.

Unemployment Supplement
Paid in certain circumstances to industrially injured pensioners, usually in place of sickness benefit.

Vehicles
A single-seat three-wheeled vehicle or ordinary four-wheeler car plus car allowance, tax, insurance and replacement are available to disabled people, if they are fit to control the vehicle and comply with certain qualifications.

War Pension
Pensions plus allowances paid to people disabled through war or armed forces service and to widows and some dependants.

Wheelchairs
May be provided for indoor or outdoor use. Home adaptations, if necessary, can be carried out.

The information division of the Department of Health and Social Security issue a booklet called *Family Benefits and Pensions* and also one called *Help for Handicapped People* which give general guidance on all Social Security benefits and the conditions for granting them. If you are severely disabled, registration on the Disabled Persons Register at the Social Services Department (although voluntary) is worth-while as it helps to ensure that care and benefits are received.

2 Employment

The Department of Employment also publish a book called *Services for the Disabled* (available from H.M.S.O., 49 High Holborn, London WC1, tel: 928 6977 – or mail order 928 1321). This book (price 70p) covers special, social and medical services and deals comprehensively with every aspect of rehabilitation, vocational training and employment of the disabled. It is necessary to contact the Disablement Resettlement Officer at your local Employment exchange in order to be included in the Disabled Persons Employment Register if you wish to take advantage of the variety of services mentioned in the D.O.E. book.

Section 2

Organisations which can help

ABBEYFIELD SOCIETY
Head Office: 35 High Street, Potters Bar, Herts
Potters Bar 43371

Local Abbeyfield societies, set up throughout the country, acquire or build houses to provide bedsitting-rooms for five to eight resident old people and accommodation for a housekeeper. Residents furnish their own rooms and each house aims to be self-supporting and achieve a family setting while preserving the privacy and independence of each resident. Local societies try to cater for local lonely old people of every background and income level. There are over 300 such societies and some 500 houses.

AGE CONCERN (England)
(National Old People's Welfare Council)
Bernard Sunley House, 60 Pitcairn Road, Mitcham, Surrey CR4 3LL
01 947 3671

A parent body which brings together in consultation national voluntary organisations working for the benefit of old people. Acts as a centure of information on all subjects regarding the welfare of old people. Welfare committees are established throughout the country to find out local needs and to help with accommodation, clubs, meals, visiting, chiropody, night attendance, group holidays and other services. Publications lists available.

AL-ANON FAMILY GROUPS U.K. AND EIRE
c/o St. Giles Centre, Camberwell Church Street, London SE5
01 703 0397

The Al-Anon family groups are nation-wide and are able to help the families of alcoholics, who can find great relief and hope in discussing their anxieties with those whose alcoholic partners have recovered. They learn that there are things which they can do directly to help themselves and, indirectly, to help their partners. (No subscription.)

ALCOHOLICS ANONYMOUS
11 Redcliffe Gardens, London SW10 9BG
01 352 9669) } *for London area only*
01 352 1626) }
01 352 9779 *for the rest of the country*

The only qualification for membership of this nation-wide society is a sincere desire to stop drinking. Attendance at one of the meetings of the 400 groups in the U.K. brings men and women into contact with others who can share their experiences and give strength and hope to each other in order to solve their common problems. (No subscription.)

ANOREXICS ANONYMOUS
21 Kitson Road, Barnes, London SW13

Formed to help people recover from *anorexia nervosa,* a nervous condition which affects the appetite and results in a dramatic loss of weight. Sympathetic advice and understanding is given to people when gaining weight during recovery.

ARTHRITIS AND RHEUMATISM COUNCIL
Faraday House, 8/10 Charing Cross Road, London WC2H 0HN
01 240 0871

This organisation finances research into the causes and treatment of rheumatism, arthritis, fibrositis and allied complaints. They also publish a booklet on gout, available through a doctor.

ASSOCIATION OF BLIND AND PARTIALLY SIGHTED STUDENTS AND TEACHERS
c/o Terry Moody, Department of Political Economy, University of Glasgow, Glasgow G12 8RT
041 339 8855 Ext. 559

The Association exists to help students through courses at Polytechnics, Universities and Colleges of Education, and to assist teachers in overcoming their handicap. It also aims to encourage the R.N.I.B. to produce more tapes and Braille books, and helps the blind student to get a job.

Association of Disabled Professionals
Longacre, Horsleys Green, High Wycombe, Bucks HP14 3UX
High Wycombe 3801
Radnage 2355 *evenings only*

The A.D.P. was formed because little of the existing rehabilitation machinery is geared to assess, train and find employment for the professional person disabled in childhood or in adult life. The Association explores special education and employment problems experienced by professionals and exists to help them to develop their physical and mental capacities to the full and to promote their entry into the professions.

Association for Speech-impaired Children
Room 11, Nuffield Centre, Swinton Street, London WC1
01 837 8855

Aims to develop understanding of speech impairment in children by supporting treatment and education, by training personnel and by promoting research. An advisory and information service is provided.

Association for Research into Restricted Growth
3 West Croft, West End, Cleveden, Bristol

Helps with advice, social contact and research into causes of dwarfism in all its forms and the social and physical disadvantages of such a condition.

Association for Spina Bifida and Hydrocephalus
Devonshire Street House, 30 Devonshire Street, London W1N 2EB
01 486 6100
01 930 9060

Seventy local associations throughout Britain provide mutual support for people suffering from this disorder by helping with equipment, grants, holidays and, in some cases, play-groups. The national organisation co-ordinates the work of the local associations and offers an information service on equipment (including toys), education, welfare, training and employment. A publications list is available.

Association to Combat *Huntington's Chorea*
45 Godmere Crescent, Ashford, Middx TW15 2DE
Ashford 50282

The Committee assists people with the disease, and their families and friends, in meeting the social, economic and emotional problems resulting from the disease. They have set up branches in major towns throughout the country and more are in formation. They publish an explanatory booklet for families and friends of patients with the disease.

Automobile Association
Fanum House, Basingstoke, Hants RG21 2EA
Basingstoke 62940

The A.A. publish a Guide for the disabled which gives detailed information on hotels, motels, guest houses and farmhouses throughout the country offering suitable accommodation for disabled people. The Guide also includes information on every point of interest to the disabled driver, from parking, toilets and car repairers to travelling on the Continent. Price 15p (free to members).

Belfast Association of the Hard of Hearing *see* British Association of the Hard of Hearing

Be Not Anxious
89 Bredhurst Road, Wigmore, Gillingham, Kent
Medway 34262

Sufferers from 'nerves', anxiety states or panic attacks (often caused by fear), are helped by phone, letter or cassette tape to understand what produces their physical symptoms. They are also told how to ease their nervous condition and control it. (No fee – just postage.)

Birth Control Campaign
233 Tottenham Court Road, London W1P 9AE
01 580 9360

A pressure group calling for comprehensive birth-control facilities (contraception, sterilisation and, where necessary, abortion) within the National Health Service, for better education in family planning and to tackle the problem of unwanted pregnancy.

B.I.T.
151 Westbourne Park Road, London W11
01 229 8219

A free, 24-hour-a-day information service (best on 'underground' activities, drugs, political and social movements). A doctor is available every Wednesday evening from 6 p.m. to give advice.

BREAK
100 First Avenue, Bush Hill Park, Enfield, Middlesex EN1 1BP
01 366 0253

Everybody needs a break and this organisation runs three holiday centres in Norfolk, for unaccompanied handicapped children. The centres are open all the year to deprived, disturbed, and maladjusted children as well as those who are physically handicapped. Children are accepted up to 15 years of age and it is occasionally possible to accommodate entire familes. Special diets are catered for and the staff includes a State Registered Nurse. Details of cost will be given on application.

BREAKTHROUGH TRUST
103 Ridgeway Drive, Bromley, Kent BR1 5DB

Through the activities of a number of groups in the country, Breakthrough brings deaf and hearing people into contact with each other. Emphasis is on monthly group meetings but there are also monthly discussion groups, a children's music group and holidays for the multi-handicapped deaf child. A wide variety of other activities are arranged by local groups and enquiries are welcome from any area.

BRITISH ASSOCIATION FOR THE RETARDED
17 Pembridge Square, London W2 4EP
01 229 1855

Primarily a pressure group to promote the interests and safeguard the statutory rights of the mentally retarded. Conferences, study tours and seminars are arranged so that all concerned with the retarded are fully informed of the most recent developments. A legal service is available together with an information and advisory service. Film programmes and exhibitions are arranged.

British Association of Retired Persons
14 Frederick Street, Edinburgh EH2 2HB
031 225 7334

Acts as a 'voice' for the older generation in Britain and its objective is to help all older and retired people to mitigate the deterioration of living standards of those on fixed or nearly fixed incomes. Despite its title, it is not necessary to be retired at the time of joining. A bulletin is published every quarter, and posted to all members, which contains particulars of political and other action taken on behalf of the retired and gives information on how members can help themselves, but individual queries cannot be answered because of staff shortage.

British Association of the Hard of Hearing
Briarfield, Syke Ungs, Iver, Bucks SL0 9ER

Belfast Association of the Hard of Hearing
2 Aragreen Crescent, Belmont, Belfast BT4 3F3

Acts as an information and advice centre to deal with all problems arising from impaired hearing and is also active in encouraging the establishment of clubs and classes throughout the country. The Association involves itself in the organisation of educational week-ends, rallies, holidays, youth activities, encouragement of the study of the arts and of the practice of lip-reading, and improvement of speech.

British Council for the Rehabilitation of the Disabled (REHAB)
Tavistock House South, Tavistock Square, London WC1H 9LB
01 387 4037

Acts as an information and advisory service in all matters concerned with the rehabilitation of the disabled. Explores ways and means of securing employment for the mentally and physically handicapped and in general acts as a central co-ordinating body for all those concerned, by whatever means, with the rehabilitation of the disabled.

British Deaf Association
38 Victoria Place, Carlisle CA1 1EX
Carlisle 20188

The B.D.A. is the national representative body for lifelong deaf people and unites them through congresses, conferences, rallies, further education, day and residential courses, summer schools and winter rallies. Grants are made to deaf people in special need and the Association runs a home for elderly and infirm men and women and arranges holidays. They publish a very comprehensive magazine, literature and documentary films helpful to the deaf.

British Dental Health Foundation
3 Harcourt House, 19a Cavendish Square, London W1
01 580 0778

Aims to promote a greater awareness of dental health to the public and to the dental profession. Is happy to give advice on dental care to private individuals.

British Diabetic Association
3–6 Alfred Place, London WC1E 7EE
01 636 7355

An organisation founded in 1934 by H. G. Wells and Dr. R. D. Lawrence (both diabetics) to provide advice and help for diabetics, to overcome prejudice and ignorance about the disease and to raise money for research towards a cure. The Association organises annual holidays for diabetic children and answers enquiries on employment, insurance, holidays, convalescent facilities, diet and cookery. It also publishes a newspaper.

British Dyslexia Association
18 The Circus, Bath, Somerset BA1 2ET
Bath 28880

Dyslexia (word blindness) is a specific disability related to reading, writing, spelling and, occasionally, arithmetic. Dyslexic children are likely to write letters the wrong way round or upside down. Spelling may be quite bizarre and bear no relationship to the sounds of the words at all. The aims of the Association are to secure recognition by Local Authorities of dyslexia as a disability; to press for adequate facilities for the diagnosis of dyslexia; to bring to the attention of all teaching staff, particularly those in primary schools, the existence of dyslexia and the importance of early recognition of the symptoms. The Association will put people in touch with their nearest group who will be able to supply book lists, journals and advice on treatment.

British Epilepsy Association
('The Candle')
3–6 Alfred Place, London WC1E 7EB
01 580 2704

Scottish Epilepsy Association
48 Govan Road, Glasgow G51 1JL
041 427 4911

A national body which aims to correct many of the misconceptions about the cause and effects of this common illness which affects one in every 200 people. The Association runs an information and advice bureau on employment, insurance, schooling, accommodation and other problems, publishes leaflets and booklets for free general distribution and raises money for research.

British Guild for Sudden Infant Death Study
28 Ty Gwyn Crescent, Penylan, Cardiff
Cardiff 35252

Founded to stimulate public awareness of 'cot deaths', and particularly to emphasise the natural, non-accidental nature of the causation. Objects are to stimulate research, bring about administrative reforms in registration and coroners' procedures and especially to contact newly bereaved parents to offer sympathy and information and to relieve the almost universal feelings of self-reproach.

British Heart Foundation
57 Gloucester Place, London W1H 4DH
01 935 0185

The Foundation's prime aim is to raise and provide money for research. Although entirely dependent on voluntary contributions, it has awarded grants to over 300 research programmes in the U.K. The Foundation publishes a number of leaflets which give advice and encouragement to someone who has had a heart attack or a stroke and other leaflets on research, drugs and other topics related to heart disease. A 16mm film is available for loan and a poster can be bought (useful for offices and factories) which illustrates how to take emergency action on heart–lung resuscitation.

British Institution of Practical Psychology
67 Highbury New Park, London N5 2EZ
01 226 3569

The slogan of the British Institute is 'Look out – not in: look up – not down!' Through a four-month postal course, giving the basic principles of a healthy mind and outlook supported by personal supervision and advice, the Institute aims to educate people to 'know themselves and then to use themselves by reconstructing and re-educating the sub-conscious mind'. And introductory booklet and the cost of the course is sent on application.

British Limbless Ex-Service Men's Association
Frankland Moore House, 185/7 High Road, Chadwell Heath, Essex RM6 6NA

Assists and advises on all matters of pensions, allowances, welfare and employment. Ensures that artificial limbs are of the best, and establishes homes for those who, having lost limbs, need special care. There are three residential convalescent homes and 113 branches of the Association throughout Britain.

British Migraine Association
6 Bryanstone Road, Bournemouth BH3 7JE
Bournemouth 59379

The pain of a migraine attack can be among the most agonising suffered by a human being. This Association, apart from acting as a pressure group to try to bring about the wider use of preventative treatments, produces regular news-letters and literature which give up-to-date information on treatments and clinics where treatment can be obtained.

British Polio Fellowship
(The Infantile Paralysis Fellowship)
Bell Close, West End Road, Ruislip, Middx HA4 6LP
Ruislip 75515

Northern Ireland Polio Fellowship
485 Antrim Poad, Belfast BT15 3BP

The Fellowship helps the 12,000 polio victims throughout the country through its personal welfare service and newsletter. The aim of the Fellowship is to rehabilitate victims of the disease and to provide educational and recreational facilities. It operates through 75 branches and has residential homes, sheltered work schemes and holiday homes.

British Red Cross Society
9 Grosvenor Crescent, London SW1
01 235 5454

The Red Cross is known throughout the world for its work in the relief of suffering. The Society is also active in service to the community in Britain by providing a wide variety of services – escorting, hospital and home visiting, shopping, meals-on-wheels, clubs, holidays, residential homes for infirm old people and the handicapped – and organises swimming, riding and other sports for the disabled.

British Rheumatism and Arthritis Association
1 Devonshire Place, London W1N 2BD
01 935 9905/6

The Association carries on a constant programme of educational films and lectures to try to break down apathy to the disease at all levels and obtain more and better facilities for early treatment. Advice is given on accommodation, holidays, aids and gadgets and grants are sometimes made. The Association runs three holiday hotels at Birchington, Kent; Poole, Dorset; and Nairn. The Association also publishes a book on gout.

BRITTLE BONE SOCIETY
63 Byron Crescent, Dundee DD3 6SS
Dundee 81130

The Society's objects are to raise funds for research into *osteogenesis imperfecta* (brittle bones) and similar disorders, and to allow patients and their relatives to get in contact with each other and exchange information. A regular newsletter is published and information given on sources of help and any welfare benefits to which sufferers may be entitled.

BROOK ADVISORY CENTRES
233 Tottenham Court Road, London W1
01 580 2991

Seven centres in Birmingham, Bristol, Cambridge, Coventry, Edinburgh, Liverpool and London specialise in providing advice on birth control and counselling on emotional and sexual problems for young people. Cyto tests, pregnancy tests and abortion counselling and referral are available. Consultation and contraceptive supplies are available free at all centres except that in Bristol.

BUCKETS AND SPADES
20 Mersham Drive, London NW9 9PN

A Jewish holiday home for mentally handicapped children of all religions. The main objective is to provide holidays and short-term care for children under the ideal conditions at the home at St. Leonards-on-Sea. Age limits are under 13 for boys and under 16 for girls. There is no charge to parents but a donation is welcome. During the first quarter of each year the home is open to handicapped adults. Applications may be made directly or through the Social Services Department of the local authority.

CAMPHILL VILLAGE TRUST
Delrow House, Hillfield Lane, Aldenham, Watford WD2 8DJ
Radlett 6006

Three villages providing general care, education and hostels in a working community for mentally handicapped adults. There is a wide range of work in the villages which includes farming, weaving, glass engraving, baking and pottery.

CANCER INFORMATION ASSOCIATION
Gloucester Green, Oxford OX1 2EQ
Oxford 46654

The Association offers free advice by telephone or at a personal visit and a film hire service. It produces a number of posters and leaflets and a concise explanatory booklet outlining the earliest symptoms of the commonest forms of cancer.

C.A.R.E.
(Cancer After-Care and Rehabilitation Society)
Lodge Cottage, Church Lane, Timsbury, Bath, Somerset BA3 1LF
Timsbury 70731

People are more frightened of cancer than of any other disease. Fear of pain, of losing loved ones, of effects on dependents, spoils the lives of many men and women. C.A.R.E. is a group of people who have all had cancer themselves and who offer optimistic advice and encouragement to those who fear they have the disease and help with rehabilitation to those who have had operations. They publish a newsletter and, if possible, will visit patients to allay fear and to give practical help and advice.

CARR-GOMM SOCIETY
36 Gomm Road, London SE16 2GX
01 237 2318

A non-denominational society which helps the lonely of all ages and both sexes through the medium of small houses and flats each containing four to seven tenants in the middle of neighbourly communities. Each tenant has a private room; there is a housekeeper in each house and the tenants pay equal shares toward total running costs. Most of the houses are in south-east London.

CARTER FOUNDATION

34 Seymour Street, London W1
01 262 6689

The foundation has established out-patient clinics to provide free medical and psychological treatment to men and women suffering from alcoholism. Patients seen by appointment.

CATHOLIC MARRIAGE ADVISORY COUNCIL

Clitherow House, 15 Lansdowne Road, London W11 3AJ
01 727 014/2

The Council arranges lectures in schools and training colleges and organises courses for engaged couples. Local centres, staffed by trained married counsellors, provide help and advice for those with marital difficulties. A medical advisory service is provided by each centre, giving advice particularly on birth regulation.

CENTRAL BUREAU FOR EDUCATIONAL VISITS AND EXCHANGES (D.I.V.E.)

43 Dorset Street, London W1H 3FN
01 486 5101

An international clearing house for information on travel and exchange opportunities for the disabled. A directory is available which gives disabled people information on a wide range of holidays abroad from winter sports in Switzerland to 'handicamping' in Greenland.

CENTRAL COUNCIL FOR THE DISABLED

34 Eccleston Square, London SW1V 1PE
01 834 0747/8

Acts for the general welfare of the disabled and as a central bureau of information on progress of work in aid of the disabled all over the world. Publishes a holiday guide and maintains an exhibition of aids. A bi-monthly journal is published.

Cheshire Foundation Homes for the Sick

7 Market Mews, London W1Y 8HP
01 499 2665

The Foundation cares for the severely disabled and chronically sick, mainly of the younger age group, for whom the hospitals can do nothing further and who have nowhere else suitable to live. Residents are admitted according to need, irrespective of race, creed or social status, and activities in the homes include typing, sewing, painting, writing, photography, ham radio, etc. Most homes can offer short holidays to disabled people.

Chest and Heart Association

Tavistock House North, Tavistock Square, London WC1H 9JE
01 387 3012
Also: N. Ireland Chest and Heart Association, 28 Bedford Street, Belfast BT2 7FE.

Publishes educational leaflets, books and manuals on diseases of the heart and chest; carries out research on education and rehabilitation for sufferers from tuberculosis and diseases of the chest and heart.

Cheyne Holiday Club for Handicapped Children

see Handicapped Adventure Playground Association

Church Army

Headquarters: 185 Marylebone Road, London NW1 5QL
01 262 3211

Social work includes men's and youths' hostels and homes; disabled men's workshops; youth centres; women's and girls' hostels; homes and flatlets for elderly people.

Church of England Children's Society
Old Town Hall, Kennington Road, London SE11 4QP
01 735 2441

Offers a comprehensive child-care service to deprived children and their families. The society has over seventy social workers. It provides counselling and grant aid to families in need, is the largest voluntary adoption agency and also arranges fostering. It runs eighty residential establishments – family homes for school-age children, nurseries, residential care for maladjusted and physically handicapped children, hostels for diabetic children, working teenagers, unsupported mothers and children; day nurseries and playgroups.

Coeliac Society of Great Britain and Northern Ireland
P.O.Box 181, London NW2 2QY

Advises on gluten-free foods, recipes, eating out, travelling, etc. There are branches in many parts of the country and members, who must be medically diagnosed coleiacs, are put in touch with one another if they wish. The Society publishes a regular newsletter, holds meetings, has published a handbook and has made a film (available from Concord Films) and an illustrated lecture-tape.

College of Speech Therapists
47 St John's Wood High Street, London NW8 7NJ
01 586 1958

The College publishes a series of pamphlets on speech therapy (the treatment of disorder, deviation, loss or partial breakdown of speech). They will also put people in need of treatment in touch with a qualified speech therapist in their area.

Colostomy Welfare Group
38/39 Eccleston Square, London SW1V 1PB
01 828 5175

Aims to help people who have undergone or are about to undergo colostomy, or similar operations, by allaying fear and anxiety and offering advice and information. The Group runs a welfare visiting service in Greater London and from seven other centres in the British Isles. A postal advice service is available for patients who live far from one of these Centres.

Community Relations Commission

15/16 Bedford Street, London WC2E 9HX
01 836 3545

The Commission's chief task is to eliminate prejudice and to encourage co-operation and understanding between different ethnic groups. The Commission provides a service of advice to the Government, to local authorities and to other statutory and voluntary organisations concerned with community relations, and it advises, assists and helps to finance community relations councils.

Community Transport

31 Poland Street, Manchester M4 6AZ
061 205 2226

Provides one of the most essential services to self-help groups – transport. The 'fleet' consists of lorries, ambulances, minibuses and a breakdown truck, all of which can be used to transport people or goods and thus assist the groups in becoming more effective in their efforts to alleviate social need.

Contact

15 Henrietta Street, Covent Garden, London WC2E 8QH
01 240 0630

Old-age and loneliness often go hand in hand and this organisation, by encouraging the setting up of independent groups throughout the country, ensures that 12 lonely old people from the same area have at least one event a month to look forward to in each other's company and in the company of 12 volunteers. On one Sunday afternoon every month the 12 volunteers (6 drivers with their own cars and 6 passenger helpers) collect the same old people and drive out to tea at the home of a host or hostess. As one London Borough alone has over 6000 lonely old people, volunteers and organisers are badly needed to set up new Contact groups.

CONTACT HOUSE
126 Blythe Road, London W14

An experimental international self-help centre for the blind, where social and educational activities take place. These activities range from concerts, hobbies and group meetings to the teaching of braille and new ventures into sound recording.

COUNCIL OF SOCIAL SERVICE FOR WALES *see* NATIONAL COUNCIL OF SOCIAL SERVICES

COURT OF PROTECTION
Staffordshire House, 25 Store Street, London WC1E 7BP
01 636 6877 Ext. 203

When a mental patient is incapable of managing his affairs, the Court of Protection (an office of the Supreme Court) deals with the protection and management of his property. Application to the Court may be made by any person (but preferably a near relative).

CRUSE
The Charter House, 6 Lion Gate Gardens, Richmond, Surrey TW9 2DF
01 940 2660

This national organisation exists to aid widows by giving practical help and encouragement in adapting to bereavement and loneliness. It also helps them in making unaccustomed and difficult decisions at a time of stress and advises on managing on a possibly lower income. In short, the group helps them to build new bridges and start again. Individual and group counselling, parents' circles and social amenities are features of the organisation's work.

CYSTIC FIBROSIS RESEARCH TRUST
5 Blyth Road, Bromley, Kent BR1 3RS
01 464 7211

The aims of the trust are to educate the public about this uncommon disease and help to promote vital early diagnosis in young children. The Trust also finances research aimed at finding a complete cure. It is establishing branches and groups throughout the U.K. for the purpose of helping and advising parents with the everyday problem of caring for children with the disease.

Depressives Anonymous

c/o Mrs. A. J. Stevenson, 19 Merley Ways, Wimbourne Minster, Dorset BH21 1QN
Wimbourne 3957

Based on the conviction that one depressive is best equipped to befriend another, the organisation acts as a 'hot line' between people who have been through, or are going through, a similar depressing experience. In particular, it can help a woman suffering from 'baby blues', a depression which, for some, lingers for a long time after the birth of a baby and seems to be entirely inexplicable. Some local groups have been formed and others are in process of formation.

Disabled Living Foundation

346 Kensington High Street, London W14 8NS
01 602 2491/5

The philosophy of the Foundation is that careful study will generally relieve bad conditions and subsequent action can often return opportunities hitherto lost to the disabled. They run an Aids Centre where all kinds of aids for the disabled can be seen, handled and demonstrated and an information service on a subscription basis covering the widest possible range of subjects concerning the lives of the disabled.

Disabled Motorists' Federation

83 Fiddlers Lane, Irlam, Manchester M30 6HN

An organisation run by the disabled for the disabled which produces a bi-monthly newsletter circulated to all members. The Federation works in the interests of disabled motorists or would-be motorists (driving tuition is given) and is involved in all community problems.

DISABLEMENT INCOME GROUP
Queens House, 180/182a Tottenham Court Road,
London W1P 0BD
01 636 1946/7

A vigorous pressure group, with more than fifty branches throughout the country, which campaigns for a National Disability Income paid as a right to all disabled people who are often forced to live below subsistence level. The D.I.G. Advisory Service, based at the London office, gives individual disabled people advice on their financial problems and is dedicated to helping them claim every benefit and aid to which they are entitled under the provisions of the statutory services. D.I.G. publishes a useful free booklet on services and general information for the disabled.

DR. BARNARDO'S
Tanner's Lane, Barkingside, Ilford, Essex
01 550 8822

Provides care and treatment, both residential and non-residential, for children in need, irrespective of creed or colour, in the 100 homes and schools in the British Isles. There is also a Family Care Service and a Family Rehabilitation Unit.

DOWNS BABIES ASSOCIATION
c/o Chairman, Quinborne Community Centre, Ridgacre Road, Birmingham B32 2TW
Harborne 1374

Membership of this Association is open to any parent of a mongol baby and the core of a very detailed course of early sensory and motor training followed by pre-school education is given by the parents for parents. Where a parent makes an approach directly to the Association the consent of the child's doctor is needed. Development assessments are carried out at two Centres in Birmingham, where individual advice is also offered.

DUET
11 Macclesfield Street, London W1V 7LF

Brings together people in London who want to meet people. There are socials in central London every weekday and Saturday evening at which there is dancing, table tennis, draughts, chess or simply the opportunity to chat over a drink and snacks at the bar. Coach trips, a group holiday scheme and a postal introduction service are all part of Duet's activities. There is a membership fee or, alternatively, an entry charge for the socials.

Duke of Edinburgh's Award Scheme
2 Old Queen Street, Westminster, London SW1H 9HR
01 930 7681

The young physically handicapped can enter for this Award for personal achievements by obtaining a Record Book from their school, youth club or organisation. They must have their parents' consent and the approval of the local doctor. Many handicapped children carry out the same programme of wide-ranging activities and meet the same requirements as able-bodied boys and girls. Appropriate adjustments are made for others to accommodate their individual handicap without lowering of standards.

Elderly Invalids Fund
10 Fleet Street, London EC4 1BB
01 353 1892

The Fund assists people who have reached or are over the age of 60 (for women) and 65 (for men) by giving financial help, information and advice. Anyone with a problem which accompanies old age can apply to them for help which can take the form of contributions towards nursing-home fees, advice on accommodation and services and help in the home, including holiday relief. The Fund will also try to suggest a likely source of help to any application whose needs are outside its own scope.

Electronic Remote Controls for the Severely Disabled
Maling P.O.S.M. Limited, St. Andrews Way Industrial Estate,
Bicester Road, Aylesbury, Bucks HP19 3AS
Aylesbury 86701/2

A small company concerned in the design, development and production of a range of control systems for the very severely disabled which help towards allowing disabled people to remain within the family circle whenever practicable.

Elizabeth Fitzroy Homes for the Handicapped Trust
The Coach House, Whitegates, Liss, Hants
Liss 3577

The Trust runs four small friendly homes for mentally and physically handicapped children; the most recent home caters for boys over 15 years. Unfortunately there is always a long waiting list, but information about the homes will be sent on request.

The Employment Fellowship
Drayton House, Gordon Street, London WC1H 0BE
01 387 1828

Sheltered work centres where elderly people can work at tasks adjusted to their strength and skill. Companionship, a useful occupation and a supplementary income are the rewards.

Eye Care Information Bureau
55 Park Lane, London W1Y 4LH
01 499 0609

Publishes educational leaflets about caring for the eyes and answers individual queries ranging from treatment (though the Bureau does not itself undertake treatment), to the fitting of contact lenses and cosmetic surgery.

Ex-Services Mental Welfare Society
37 Thurloe Street, London SW7 2LL
01 584 8688

Ex-Services Mental Welfare Society – Scottish Office
Baltic Chambers, 3 Cadogan Street, Glasgow G2 6QE
041 221 1303

The Society exists to assist ex-members of the Forces, including the Merchant Navy, who are suffering from nervous or mental disabilities arising from active or long regular service. It has access to consultant psychiatrists in every county and maintains its own treatment centre, old people's home and large industrial centre where patients unable to face competitive life may work and live under sheltered conditions.

Families Need Fathers
23 Holmes Road, London NW5
01 242 1860

A group of divorced men and sympathetic women who are attempting to promote the rights and needs of fathers excluded from the family by a divorce which has granted custody of the children to the mother.

Family Planning Association
Margaret Pyke House, 27/35 Mortimer Street, London 1WA 4QW
01 636 7866

Aims to educate the public to take personal responsibility in sexual relationships and to prevent the poverty, hardship and distress caused by unwanted pregnancies. Over 1000 clinics of the F.P.A. give medical advice and assistance with contraception, involuntary sterility, and with difficulties in marriage. Mail order sales of contraceptives and books and free information leaflets are available. There are 12 Youth Advisory centres which cater especially for young people over 16.

Family Service Units
207 Old Marylebone Road, London NW1 5QP
01 402 5175

Dedicated to undertake intensive and comprehensive welfare work among families who are unable to maintain proper standards of home and child care without special assistance. There are 19 units spread over the country.

Federation of Mental Patients' Unions
37 Mayola Road, Clapton, London E5
01 986 5251

Represents mental patients wherever they need to be represented. Seeks to inform patients and ex-patients about their rights, especially the right to appeal against compulsory detention. Membership is open to any person who is or has been an in-patient, day-patient or out-patient in any mental hospital, or a patient under psychiatric care elsewhere.

Finchale Training College
Finchale, Durham.
Durham 62634

A residential college which provides training for disabled men and women over the age of 16 in a variety of occupations including gardening, typewriter mechanics, watch and clock repair, carpentry, servicing of domestic electrical appliances, general office practice and machine operation.

Friedrich's Ataxia Group
Bolsover House, 5/6 Clipstone Street, London W1
01 636 2042
Also: Cambusnethan, Tillietudlem, Nr. Lesmahagow, Strathclyde, Scotland

Supported by doctors, social workers, parents and friends of sufferers of this very rare disease (which usually manifests itself at puberty), the aim of the group is to make available as much information as possible about the disease, the cause of which is unknown. They publish a useful booklet which outlines some of the common problems encountered by people with the disease and they give practical advice about how these problems may be tackled. The group also organises fund-raising activities to enable more research to be carried out.

Friend

47 Church Street, London NW8
01 402 6750 *7.30 p.m. – 9.30 p.m. only*

A service intended to help men and women with problems relating to homosexuality, which can include acute loneliness, conflict with the law and religious conflict, and the difficulties which arise from being 'different' in a society which demands conformity and often imposes on homosexuals the need to lead a double life.

Friends International Centre

Courtauld House, Torrington Place, London WC1E 7JJ
01 387 5648 *office*
01 387 3669 *visitors*

A self-help community established by the Friends Service Council, a Quaker body. The centre extends a welcome to members, residents and overnight visitors (who need not be members). Membership is open to anyone for a small subscription and entitles the member to use all the facilities of the centre, including cheap accommodation, meals, laundry, study room, craft room, etc. There is also a consultancy service for (or about) students and non-students both from Britain and overseas and advice is available on all matters of particular interest to them.

Friends of the Elderly and Gentlefolk's Help

42 Ebury Street, London SW1
01 730 8263

Gives general financial help to the elderly and disabled of all classes. The Society cares for elderly gentlefolk in thirteen residential homes with nursing wings attached and often makes regular allowances to the elderly to help with private old people's homes or nursing-home fees.

Gamblers Anonymous
17/23 Blantyre Street, Cheyne Walk, London SW10
01 353 3060 }
01 654 3276 } *home numbers*
01 722 8661 }

The work of this organisation (which has over 30 groups throughout the country) is based on group therapy, and is aimed at helping the compulsive gambler who, like the alcoholic, leaves a trail of broken homes, broken hearts and bad debts behind him or her. Practical help and advice in solving immediate problems is given to each new member and the partner or parent of the gambler is also encouraged to attend GAM-ANON in order that they should be able to work together to fight this compulsion.

Gingerbread
9 Poland Street, London W1Z 3DZ
01 734 9014

An association for one-parent families. The association gives sympathy and encouragement, by telephone and correspondence, to parents who are divorced, separated, widowed or unmarried, and to those whose partners are in prison, in hospital or are seriously disabled. Regular group meetings are arranged and information sheets are available on a variety of topics ranging from legal rights to holiday advice. The association also aims to draw attention to inadequate provision in the law and social services for such families.

Girl Guides Association
17/19 Buckingham Palace Road, London SW1W 0PT
01 834 6242

The Extension Group provides a place in the Girl Guides Association for every handicapped girl (Brownies 7–11, Guides 10–16, Rangers from 14) who understands the Promise and wishes to join. Through the Extension Group, which includes girls who are not handicapped, a disabled or mentally handicapped girl not only gains personal skill, but finds adventure, fun, friendship and opportunities for service to others. There is guiding for the deaf and the blind as well, and girls can join a pack even if they are in hospital or homebound.

GRACE
Leigh Corner, Leigh Hill Road, Cobham, Surrey KT1 2HW
Cobham 2928

A free, residential advisory service for the elderly covering the South of England (but excluding Greater London). Detailed information concerning privately run nursing homes, some hotels and guest houses is available, together with up-to-date information on vacancies. Fifteen area visitors visit all the accommodation offered and keep the information concerning them up-to-date.

GUIDE DOGS FOR THE BLIND ASSOCIATION
113 Uxbridge Road, Ealing, London W5 5TQ
01 567 7001

The Association aims to provide blind adults with a guide dog and to train dogs and owners together. They have centres at Bolton, Exeter, Forfar and Leamington Spa, where dogs are trained and blind persons spend four weeks in residential accommodation when they are being trained with their guide dogs. There is an age restriction of 18 to 60 years for new blind applicants, but the Association will always consider people over 60 if they can really benefit from having a guide dog.

GUIDEPOSTS TRUST
Marlborough Lane, Witney, Oxon.
Witney 3981/2

At the end of 1971 there were about 106,000 mentally ill patients in hospitals in England and Wales. Guideposts Trust has been established to try to set up Christian community facilities for the mentally ill, thus relieving pressure on hospitals. They plan to establish Halfway Homes for people coming out of psychiatric hospitals and Stress Centres where people can come and talk out their problems. A bi-monthly inter-denominational magazine *Guideposts* is published.

Haemophilia Society
P.O. Box 9, 16 Trinity Street, London SE1 1DE
01 407 1010

The Society exists to provide a fellowship for haemophiliacs and to give advice on their problems. It also promotes the study of the causes and treatment of haemophilia and gathers and distributes information useful to them and to the general public.

Handicapped Adventure Playground Association
2 Paultons Street, London SW3
01 352 6890
01 352 2062

Cheyne Holiday Clubs for Handicapped Children
61 Cheyne Walk, Chelsea, London SW3

'Going out to play' for severely disabled children is impossible and it was for this reason that Holiday Clubs were started. The Association provides, through the medium of play, for children and young people with mental, physical or emotional handicaps, including those of vision, hearing and perception. The four now in existence in London (Chelsea, Roehampton, Tulse Hill and Islington) provide a variety of activities for children between 7–16 for one or two whole days of each week of the holidays. Helpers, drivers and people to set up clubs in other areas are needed.

Handicapped Children's Pilgrimage Trust
95 Carshalton Road, Sutton, Surrey
01 643 4431/2

The Trust takes handicapped children between the ages of 7 to 18 on a week's pilgrimage and holiday to Lourdes immediately after Easter. The children are not housed in hospitals but in family hotels and during the week they go everywhere possible including up into the mountains. Any physically handicapped child (including non-Catholics) is eligible.

THE HOWARD LEAGUE FOR PENAL REFORM
125 Kennington Park Road, London SE11 4JP
01 735 3773

A watch-dog group which is concerned with the operation of the penal system. It particularly concerns itself with inappropriate penalties which seem likely to hinder rehabilitation; with prison conditions, and prisoners' rights, and with cases where inadequate resources are devoted to the more desirable features of the system, such as education of prisoners, after-care and probation. The Howard League also acts as a pressure group and encourages the formation of local groups where members can undertake their own investigations into conditions in prisons, detention centres and hostels in their areas, and publicise their work locally.

ILEOSTOMY ASSOCIATION OF GREAT BRITAIN AND IRELAND
Drove Cottage, Fuzzy Drove, Kempshott, Basingstoke, Hants
Basingstoke 21288

An association which gives help, encouragement and advice to people about to undergo, or who have undergone, this operation in order that they may help each other to continue their lives as normally as possible after the operation.

IN TOUCH
10 Norman Road, Sale, Cheshire M33 3DP

Puts parents who are caring for a mentally handicapped child or adult in touch with others similarly placed. They correspond and/or meet to give mutual support and exchange ideas. There is a quarterly newsletter and outgrown equipment is offered for sale. Literature is available.

INVALID CHILDREN'S AID ASSOCIATION
126 Buckingham Palace Road, London SW1 9SB
01 730 9891

When I.C.A.A. was formed nearly 80 years ago, its purpose was to arrange for 'a friend for every invalid child'. That is still the main task, although the original volunteer 'friend' has disappeared, to be replaced by highly qualified home visitors, who advise upon the care of the invalid child in the home and act as a bridge between the medical world and home. The extra cost of caring for a sick child often creates difficulties and in these cases I.C.A.A. arranges for assistance.

THE JACK HAWKINS CLUB
Greenwich District Hospital, Vanbrugh Hill, London SE10 9HE
01 858 8141

Aims to make contact with all patients who have lost their larynx through a laryngectomy operation and have therefore lost the natural means of producing speech. The Club provides a social focus and a relaxed atmosphere in which patients whose rehabilitation has been a success can give moral support and practical advice to others who have not managed to achieve a good 'pseudo voice'. Any laryngectomy patient is eligible to join and there are two other similar clubs:

'Swallow Club'
Miss J. Cooke,
Royal National E.N.T. Hospital
Gray's Inn Road, London WC1
01 837 8855

Miss V. Boby,
Speech Therapist,
New Charing Cross Hospital,
Fulham Palace Road, London SW3
01 836 7788

JEWISH AGED NEEDY PENSION SOCIETY
59 Valley Drive, Kingsbury NW9
01 204 5050

Gives pensions to indigent Jews of 60 and over through a weekly allowance.

JEWISH BLIND SOCIETY
1 Craven Hill, London W2 3EW
01 262 3111

The Society ministers to the needs of all the Jewish blind throughout the U.K. They carry out extensive welfare work and have four homes, two of which are also holiday homes. Volunteers transcribe extracts from the *Jewish Chronicle* and other articles of Jewish interest for weekly circulation to members.

JOHN GROOM'S ASSOCIATION FOR THE DISABLED
10 Gloucester Drive, London N4
01 802 7271

Provides housing and employment for the disabled, and homes for deprived able-bodied children and elderly females. There are two sheltered workshops at Edgware with homes nearby and a home for deprived children in Kent. The Association also runs a convalescent holiday home for children in Essex.

JOINT COMMITTEE ON MOBILITY FOR THE DISABLED
Wanborough Manor, Wanborough, Guildford, Surrey
Guildford 810484

A representative body of member and observer organisations which exists to pool expert specialised knowledge on mobility for the disabled. The J.C.M.D. ensures that the special needs of all types of disabled people are considered and that the knowledge and experience of one organisation is readily available to another. They also act as a pressure group on the Health Service to ensure awareness not only of the needs of the disabled in respect of parking concessions, road use, ramps, etc., but also of new wheelchair designs, improved invalid vehicles, hand control systems and children's aids. Help can often be obtained from the J.C.M.D. when other means of obtaining relief from statutory bodies has been exhausted, and where it is thought that there is a case for altering existing regulations.

Joint Council for the Education of Handicapped Children
4 Old Croft Road, Walton-on-the-Hill, Stafford ST17 0LS
Stafford 61108

A parent body which brings together those associations concerned with the education of all handicapped children, whether the handicap be physical, mental or emotional. The Council will direct queries to the organisation within its framework which can best answer educational questions related to the disability of each individual child.

La Leche League
48 Clarke Street, Market Harborough, Leics
Market Harborough 5937

An organisation which teaches, encourages and gives moral support to those mothers-to-be who want to breast-feed their babies.

Lady Hoare Trust for Thalidomide and other Physically Disabled Children
2 Milford House, 7 Queen Anne Street, London W1M 9FD
01 637 1545

The Trust was founded after a national appeal for children damaged by the drug thalidomide had been launched, but now looks after other physically disabled children. It has a comprehensive welfare system, employing twenty-two fully qualified medical social workers who visit and look after families under their care throughout the U.K.

Leukaemia Society
28 Eastern Road, East Finchley, London N2
01 883 4703

A group with branches throughout the country which offers friendship and understanding to sufferers of this disease and those concerned for their health. It also offers practical help with baby-minding and care of children during extended periods, help with transport and information on the most up-to-date treatment.

London Council for the Welfare of Women and Girls
16 Great Russell Street, London WC1
01 580 0478

Provides an information service on residential accommodation in the Greater London area. In addition, help and advice are available about social clubs, employment and 'au pair' agencies. Organised by the Young Women's Christian Association.

Lord Mayor Treloar Trust
Froyle Alton, Hants
Bentley 3248

The Trust runs two schools for physically handicapped children, The Lord Mayor Treloar College (for boys) and the Florence Treloar School (for girls). The College accepts boys from the age of 10, and the School is one of the few boarding schools in the country able to offer a broad secondary education to G.C.E. 'A' Level for severely disabled girls.

Louise Buchannan Memorial Fund
22 Anterberry Road, London SW20

A fund which is run voluntarily on behalf of sufferers from Hodgkin's Disease, in order to raise money to send doctors to America to learn more about the disease, which has become curable only over the last five years.

Marie Curie Memorial Foundation
124 Sloane Street, London SW1X 9BP
01 730 9157

This Foundation has twelve homes throughout the U.K. devoted solely to the care of cancer patients. They also run an area welfare and night nursing scheme to assist patients in their own homes and an education department which provides information on request. A publications list is available.

MEDIC-ALERT FOUNDATION
9 Hanover Street, London W1R 9HF
01 499 2261

The Foundation provides a bracelet or necklet with a medical insignia on one side and the appropriate medical warning on the other, with serial number, for any person with a hidden medical problem. This emblem gives an immediate warning to hospitals, doctors, police or others who might attend them at a time when they are unable to speak for themselves, such as an accident. A central file is kept in London and emergency information can be obtained by a doctor or other authorised person by making a reversed-charge telephone call from anywhere in the world. The telephone is manned day and night.

MENTAL AFTER-CARE ASSOCIATION
Eagle House, 110 Jermyn Street, London SW1Y 6HB
01 839 5953

This Association assists general hospitals and clinics with early treatment of mental and nervous disorders by providing periods of rest, or holidays, housing and rehabilitation for patients discharged from mental hospitals. It also provides long-term accommodation under supervision for certain mentally disabled people and holidays for those still under treatment.

MIGRAINE TRUST
23 Queen Square, London, WC1N 3AY
01 278 2676

Exists primarily to research into the causes of migraine, its alleviation and treatment. Up-to-date information is available on the latest discoveries for the treatment of the complaint.

MIND
(National Association for Mental Health)
22 Harley Street, London W1N 2ED
01 637 0741

SCOTTISH ASSOCIATION FOR MENTAL HEALTH
57 Melville Street, Edinburgh EH3 7HL
031 225 7632

NORTHERN IRELAND ASSOCIATION FOR MENTAL HEALTH
Beacon House, University Street, Belfast BT7 7HE
Belfast 28474/5

MIND
(National Association for Mental Health)
9a Castle Street, Cardiff
Cardiff 390950

The Association runs a walk-in advisory case work service, staffed by trained social workers to advise on the variety of problems that can arise in connection with mental ill-health. N.A.M.H. runs a holiday home for mentally subnormal patients, a home for elderly women patients, two community homes for girls needing psychiatric treatment, two special boarding schools for maladjusted children and hostels for educationally subnormal school leavers. A publications list is available.

MULTIPLE SCLEROSIS ACTION GROUP
(A.R.M.S.)
71 Gray's Inn Road, London WC1X 8TR
01 568 2255

Founded in 1974 to apply pressure for more research into the cause, cure and prevention of this disease. The group has set up a nationwide counselling service for MS suffers and their relatives, which is manned 24 hours a day, 7 days a week by MS sufferers.

MULTIPLE SCLEROSIS SOCIETY OF GREAT BRITAIN AND N. IRELAND
4 Tachbrook Street, London SW1
01 834 8231

Roosevelt Memorial (Polio) Fund
113 Vincent Street, Glasgow C2
Northern Ireland branch: 12 Lansdowne Road,
Belfast BT15 4DA

Organises the formation of local groups throughout the U.K. which give mutual help and comradeship and bring interest and hope into the lives of MS sufferers. The groups assist them with their problems and advise on how best to live within the limits of their disabilities.

Muscular Dystrophy Group of Great Britain
26 Borough High Street, London SE1 9QG
01 407 5116

The Group's objectives are to raise funds for research into the cause and cure of this disease and to give assistance to sufferers and the people who care for them.

Myasthenia Gravis Branch of the Muscular Dystrophy Group
26 Borough High Street, London SE1 9QG
01 407 5116

The Organisation has two aims – the welfare of myasthenics and fund raising. The very name and rarity of Myasthenia Gravis (serious muscle weakness) has built up a mystique about the disease, creating for the myasthenic a terrible loneliness and isolation and, even more important, a lack of understanding. The Branch has now embarked upon the task of forming local associations throughout the country in an attempt to unify the resources of Myasthenics, to provide opportunities for them and their families to meet as often as possible and to help find cause of and cure for the disease.

N.A.C.R.O.
(National Association for the Care and Resettlement of Offenders)
125 Kennington Park Road, London SE11
01 735 1151

S.A.C.R.O.
(Scottish Association for the Care and Resettlement of Offenders
1 Strathmore House, East Kilbride, Glasgow GY4 1LF

The Association concerns itself with the prevention of crime, and the care, including after-care, of offenders. It co-ordinates the work of voluntary agencies active in this field with that of statutory and other voluntary social services. A directory of organisations and projects in this work is published.

NATIONAL ASSOCIATION FOR DEAF, BLIND, AND RUBELLA CHILDREN
61 Senneleys Park Road, Northfield, Birmingham 31

Concerned with children who have difficulty with hearing, seeing and understanding. The Association gives advice, helps parents of such children to get in touch with each other, lends equipment and toys and makes money grants for special purposes.

NATIONAL ASSOCIATION FOR GIFTED CHILDREN
27 John Adam Street, London WC2N 6HX
01 839 1861/2

Gifted children are often intellectually superior to their parents, teachers and contemporaries and many have great educational and social problems. This Association acts as a centre for the collection and dissemination of information and advice relating to their needs. It also provides a meeting place for parents who can consult specialists in educational matters. There are groups throughout the country.

NATIONAL ASSOCIATION FOR THE WELFARE OF CHILDREN IN HOSPITAL
Exton House, 7 Exton Street, London SE1 8VE
01 261 1783

An Association originally formed by a group of mothers who campaigned for the right to be with their children as much as possible when they are in hospital. Now nationwide, the N.A.W.C.H. aims are summed up as follows: to bring to public notice the special needs of children in hospital, to see that new hospitals are designed with adequate accommodation for mothers and their children, to promote the treatment of sick children at home whenever possible and to assist mothers by providing details of visiting facilities in children's wards throughout the country.

National Association of Hospital Broadcasting Organisations
255 Greenside, Euxton, Chorley, Lancs PR7 6BL
Chorley 6029

There are over 190 hospital radio stations in the country, ranging from one-woman stations to highly organised complexes. All of them have the same aim, however – to entertain and inform hospital patients, to cheer them up when they're depressed, to make them smile. In the hospitals which have their own station patients can ask for record requests and birthday announcements, relatives can broadcast messages and local and hospital news is broadcast. Talking magazine and newspaper services are being started by a few hospital broadcasting stations which provide a recorded programme of news and information for blind people and others who are not able to read for themselves.

National Association of Prison Visitors
47 Hartington Street, Bedford MK41 7RN
Bedford 596763

Co-ordinates activities of unofficial visitors to H.M. prisons in England and Wales (both men's and women's prisons). Prison visitors are appointed by the prison department not the Association, but in practice most of them join the Association, which also acts as an official medium of communication in all matters concerning the welfare of the prisoner.

National Centre for Brain Damaged Children
85 Home Road, Solihull, Warwicks
Solihull 5377

An assessment centre where a child with brain damage is put on a course of home treatment (based on the Doman/Delacato method) tailored to his needs. The theory behind the treament is that there are billions of brain cells of which only a fraction are used. Even after severe brain injury not all cells are dead and the aim of the treatment is to stimulate existing cells to take over the work of dead ones. Although the centre is non-profit-making, a fee is charged to cover expenses and details of this can be obtained on application.

National Childbirth Trust
9 Queensborough Terrace, London W2 3TB
01 229 9319

The Trust's teachers prepare expectant parents for childbirth. Ante-natal classes and film shows are held at Trust headquarters and in many other areas. The Trust co-ordinates research, information and experience relevant to preparation for childbirth and publishes books and pamphlets for teachers and parents.

National Citizens' Advice Bureaux Council
26 Bedford Square, London WC1
01 636 4066

There are over 500 Bureaux in the U.K. where accurate and skilled information may be obtained on the many problems that arise in daily life, specifically relating to legislation and the use of services provided by the State. The Bureaux will also direct the citizen to the appropriate source of further specialist advice on any topic.

National Council for Civil Liberties
186 King's Cross Road, London WC1X 9DE
01 278 4575

An independent voluntary organisation protecting individual civil liberties and the rights of political, religious, racial and other minorities in Britain. It deals with such issues as the right of privacy, the treatment of gypsies, immigration and race relations, censorship, police powers and freedom of expression and association.

National Council for One-parent Families
255 Kentish Town Road, London, NW5
01 267 1361

Provides understanding, help and guidance to single mothers and their families and encourages concern of the fathers. The organisation offers an advisory service for social workers and financial help for immediate needs.

National Council for the Single Woman and Her Dependants
166 Victoria Street, London SW1E 5BR
01 828 5511

Many single women have or have had the care of elderly or infirm dependants and this can create difficulties for both the woman who may have to go out to work and the elderly relative who has to be left at home. The Council aims to set up sheltered housing, to help with holiday relief and a sitter-in service, and generally to give advice and help to women with this special problem.

National Council of Social Service
26 Bedford Square, London WC1B 3HU
01 636 4066

Scottish Council of Social Service
18/19 Claremont Crescent, Edinburgh EH7 4HX
031 556 3882

Council of Social Service for Wales
2 Cathedral Road, Cardiff CF1 9XR
Cardiff 21456

Northern Ireland Council of Social Service
2 Annandale Avenue, Belfast BT7 3JH
Belfast 643886/645489

The central agency for the co-ordination and promotion of the social services. Acts as a clearing house of information on both statutory and voluntary social services.

National Council on Alcoholism
Hope House, 45 Great Peter Street, Westminster,
London SW1P 3LT
01 222 1056/7

Alcoholism is a major cause of premature death and the National and Regional Councils offer early diagnosis of incipient alcoholism and advice on how to combat it. The Council also aims to inform the public about the disease in order to stimulate a social awareness for the need for adequate treatment and aftercare. (No subscription.)

National Deaf–Blind Helpers' League
Market Chambers, Cathedral Square, Peterborough
Peterborough 65740

The League performs a dual role in helping to inform public opinion about the problems arising from this double handicap and in bringing the deaf–blind together by letter and through the League's own magazine which is printed in braille and letterpress. They also provide help for holidays, and equipment and there is a rehabilitation centre, Rainbow Court, in Peterborough.

National Deaf Children's Society
31 Gloucester Place, London, W1H 4EA
01 486 3251

Gives personal advice to parents on early training, education and employment of their deaf children. Grants are sometimes made towards the purchase of hearing aids. Literature is available.

National Elfrida Rathbone Society
17 Victoria Park Square, Bethnal Green, London E2
01 980 4204

Provides clubs, playgroups and holiday play schemes for educationally subnormal children. There are several groups throughout the country.

National Federation of the Blind of the United Kingdom
20 Cannon Close, Raynes Park, London SW20

The Federation is run entirely by the blind, although sighted associates are welcomed. It acts as a pressure group on behalf of the blind in general and its members in particular. Among the achievements of the N.F.B. are arrangements with Wolsey Hall, Oxford, for blind people to take the College's courses (provided they have access to a tape recorder and can supply answers either in typescript or manuscript), and airline concessions whereby blind people and their guides can obtain two tickets for the price of one if the journey is for the purpose of business or other commitments.

National Federation of Claimants' Unions
19 Rea Tower, New Town, Mosborough Crescent,
Birmingham B19 3AU
021 455 0566

Established to ensure that people get their rights within the welfare state. They advise on how to deal with officials and will sometimes accompany people to appeal tribunals. There are many Claimants' Unions throughout the country and their addresses can be found through the Citizen's Advice Bureaux or by writing to the National Federation.

National Federation of Clubs for the Divorced and Separated
13 High Street, Little Shelford, Cambridge
Shelford 2544

An urgent need for divorced or separated people is the opportunity to meet others, to do something other than housework, caring for children or propping up a bar. The Federation aims to encourage individuals to start and maintain clubs all over Britain for people who know something of the loneliness that divorce or separation brings about. Besides providing a social outlet, the atmosphere of a club, where all members know something of the same dehumanising experience, can provide a background against which each sees his own position with greater objectivity and individual problems become matters of general concern.

NATIONAL FEDERATION OF 18-PLUS GROUPS
16/18 High Street, Dartford, Kent
Dartford 23591

18-plus is the natural follow-up to the Youth Club movement and is the only independent national body for people between the ages of 18 and 30. There are over 200 groups throughout the country which offer an enormous range of activities, including weekly recreational or educational meetings, usually in a pub. Weekend activities are popular and there are dances, concerts, folk evenings, night exercises with the Army, dinners, etc. There is also National Charities Week when all members are asked to help with the many projects organised. As 18-plus say of themselves: 'The list of what we get up to is infinite, and, in some cases, unprintable!'

NATIONAL FEDERATION OF EX-FAR EASTERN PRISONERS OF WAR AND CIVIL INTERNEES OF GREAT BRITAIN AND NORTHERN IRELAND
8 Lower Grosvenor Place, London SW3

During captivity in Japanese hands, many prisoners of war suffered considerably from the combined effects of malnutrition, tropical disease, ill-treatment and severe mental stress. It was not until some years after the war ended that it was noted there was a high incidence of sickness among former Japanese POWs. Because of difficulties in proving the cause of sickness so long after the event, many claimants for disablement and other benefits, and their widows, found it extremely hard to prove their case and were often refused assistance. The National Federation came into being to protect their interests by directing ex-POWs to Tropical Units for medical assessment, representing them on tribunals, giving them advice on all matters relating to pensions, education, school clothing, careers and on matters of general welfare. Applicants can be visited at home as well as helped by telephone or letter. There are branches of the Federation all over Britain.

THE NATIONAL FEDERATION OF SOLO CLUBS
851 Old Lode Lane, Solihull, Warwickshire
021 743 4133

The country's largest organisation which brings together lonely people and their children. There are 130 branches throughout the

U.K. which organise weekly socials, dancing, theatre parties, coach trips, bowling, bingo and free outings and parties for the children. The very small membership fee includes contributions to a Benevolent Fund and free insurance scheme and enables members to go on 'friendship holidays'. The Federation publishes a very helpful booklet called *Facing Life Alone.*

NATIONAL FUND FOR RESEARCH INTO CRIPPLING DISEASES
(Action Research for the Crippled Child)
Vincent House, 1 Springfield Road, Horsham, Sussex RH12 2PN

Promotes and finances research into the causes, prevention, cure and treatment of all crippling diseases. Relies on voluntary donations.

NATIONAL LEAGUE FOR THE BLIND AND DISABLED
262 Langham Road, London N15 3NS
01 888 5980

A trade union formed in 1899 by blind people to secure improvements in education and the economic and social conditions of blind and disabled people. Membership is open to any registered blind, partially blind or partially sighted person over the age of 16, and any severely disabled sighted person being trained or employed in workshops for the blind.

NATIONAL LIBRARY FOR THE BLIND
35 Great Smith Street, London SW1
01 222 2725

A comprehensive library for the blind, founded in 1882.

NATIONAL LISTENING LIBRARY
49 Great Cumberland Place, London W1H 7LH
01 723 5008/9
01 402 8380

Anyone who is unable to read books in the normal manner (other than registered blind people), is eligible to join the Library. The aim is to supply 'Talking Books', that is to say, tape cartridges and the reproducers on which to play them, for all Britain's handicapped people. The titles of cartridges range through the classics to all types of fiction from romances to thrillers, as well as works on politics, archaeology, history, biography, philosophy, sport, religion, etc. Details of cost of reproducer and tapes and how the system works can be otained on application.

NATIONAL MARRIAGE GUIDANCE COUNCIL
Herbert Gray College, Little Church Street, Rugby,
Warwicks CV21 3AP
Rugby 73241

SCOTTISH MARRIAGE GUIDANCE COUNCIL
58 Rawderston Place, Edinburgh EH12 5AZ
031 225 5006

Aims to promote successful marriage and family life. About 120 local marriage guidance councils are co-ordinated by the Council and qualified counsellers will advise on any problems creating disharmony in marriage.

NATIONAL SOCIETY FOR AUTISTIC CHILDREN
1a Golders Green Road, London NW11 8EA
01 458 4375

The society runs an advisory service for parents to help them with educational or hospital placement, and three schools, two of which are day and weekly boarding and the third fully residential. Local societies affiliated with the National Society also have schools of their own. Publications list available.

NATIONAL SOCIETY FOR CANCER RELIEF
Michael Sobell House, 30 Dorset Square, London NW1 6QL
01 402 8125

Assists cancer sufferers in financial need by grants of cash for extra food, for fuel, clothing, bedding and special equipment, grants towards nursing and convalescent home fees or day and night nursing at home and grants towards fares for those visiting patients in hospital. No genuine case has ever been refused assistance.

National Society for Mentally Handicapped Children
Pembridge Hall, 17 Pembridge Square, London W2 4EP
01 229 8941
01 727 0536

Scottish Society for Mentally Handicapped Children
69 West Regent Street, Glasgow C2

Nationally and regionally (with 400 local societies), this organisation supports parents under stress who are coping with mentally handicapped children. Welfare and counselling, speech and physiotherapy advice is given and pilot schemes in the fields of education, training and the employment of the mentally handicapped are initiated. A publications list is available.

National Society for Phenylketonuria and Allied Disorders
6 Rawdon Close, Palace Fields, Runcorn, Cheshire
Runcorn 65081

Children suffering from the dietary condition of phenylketonuria (PKU), and their parents, are helped by this society to overcome the difficulties they have in obtaining the necessary special foods. Parents of PKU children can telephone or write to the society for help and advice and personal visits can be arranged from parents of another PKU child. The society is particularly willing to help parents of newly-born children who are informed that their child has PKU.

National Society for the Prevention of Cruelty to Children
1 Riding House Street, London W1P 8AA
01 580 8812

Exists to help any child in this country whatever his colour, nationality or religion, and parents with a problem concerning the welfare of their children. The Society works with families in their own homes, striving always to keep the family together. It investigates reports of neglect or ill-treatment of children.

NEUROTICS NOMINÉ
B.C.M. Box 24, London WC1

A group run by the Marlborough Day Hospital, Hampstead, to help patients who have suffered from neuroses to solve their problems in voluntary group discussions.

NEW HORIZON
1 Macklin Street, London WC2
01 242 0010

A day centre and hostel which provides help and information for young people adrift in the West End of London. Many young people come to London from the provinces seeking jobs that do not exist and despair soon sets in. New Horizon Youth Centre acts as a referral agency by directing young people to the right sources of assistance. The Centre is also a meeting place where constructive work can be done, meals cooked, etc. Hostel accommodation is found where necessary.

NEW LIFE FOUNDATION TRUST
13 London Road, Bromley BR1 1DE
Postal address: P.O. Box 20, Bromley BR1 1DW Kent
01 460 0500

Helps people formerly addicted to drugs to find complete freedom from dependence on them. Educational books and pamphlets on the abuse of drugs are published by a department of the Trust and staff members visit schools, colleges and other establishments to lecture to both staff and students.

NORTHERN IRELAND ASSOCIATION FOR MENTAL HEALTH *see* MIND

NORTHERN IRELAND COUNCIL OF SOCIAL SERVICE *see* NATIONAL COUNCIL OF SOCIAL SERVICES

Northern Ireland Polio Fellowship *see* British Polio Fellowship

Norwood Homes for Jewish Children
74a Charlotte Street, London W1
01 636 1644

Provides homes for boys and girls of mixed ages and after-care for children who have been residents. Help is also given to families with problems concerning the welfare of children in their own homes. The Committee deals with behaviour problems of adolescent boys and girls and works with the unmarried mother and her child.

Outset
30 Craven Street, London WC2
01 930 4255

Outset is always interested in hearing from people who may wish to give some of their time to help others. They are a community work organisation which mobilises volunteers to undertake a wide range of work including decorating for old and disabled people, gardening, survey work, building adventure playgrounds and conservation work. Outset also works in co-operation with Local Authorities, helping them to locate chronically sick and disabled people who may be eligible for services under the 1970 Chronically Sick and Disabled Persons Act. Activities are not limited to London.

Over-Forty Association for Women Workers
Grosvenor Gardens House, 35/37 Grosvenor Gardens,
London SW1W 0BS
01 834 0733

This Association aims to help older women on their own in London to find suitable accommodation and employment. It provides flatlets at very modest rents, gives advice to older women seeking employment and, where possible, puts applicants in touch with likely employers.

Papworth Village Settlement
Papworth Hall, Papworth Everard, Cambridge CB3 8RF
Cambridge 088341

The settlement provides a wide range of workshop activities and suitable accommodation for single or married people suffering from most of today's more prevalent physical handicaps.

Parent to Parent Information on Adoption (P.P.I.A.S.)
26 Belsize Grove, London NW3
01 722 5328

There are 6000 children in institutions because parents can't or won't look after them, and two-thirds of all children coming into care remain in care until they are 18. Yet every adoption agency has a list of parents waiting for a child. A great many of the children are 'hard-to-place'. They may be of mixed race, or have a mental or physical handicap, or a combination of all three, yet there are many prospective parents willing and eager to give one of these children a home. P.P.I.A.S. provides such prospective parents with information on how they can set about this.

Parents Without Partners Inc
c/o 26 Bedford Square, London WC1 3HU
International H.Q.: 7910 Woodmont Avenue.
Washington DC 20014, U.S.A.

An international, non-sectarian, non-profit-making educational organisation devoted to the welfare of single parents and their children. Monthly meetings are held; an accommodation and jobs register is kept; single parents are helped to take a holiday and, in some cases, free legal advice is given. All P.W.P. members have experienced the despair and discouragement that accompany the loss of a partner and are therefore uniquely equipped to help each other in the struggle to re-establish a new kind of life.

PARKINSON'S DISEASE SOCIETY OF THE U.K.
81 Queens Road, London SW19 8NR
01 946 2500

The Society publishes a very useful and informative booklet on the disease and they maintain an information and advisory service to help patients and their relatives with problems in the home arising from Parkinson's Disease.

PATIENTS ASSOCIATION
335 Gray's Inn Road, London WC1X 8PX
01 837 7241

The Association aims to represent and further the interests of patients. It examines complaints, makes enquiries and answers queries of all kinds relating to the health service; gives information and advice; publishes leaflets to assist and inform patients.

POSSUM USERS' ASSOCIATION
25 Worlds End Lane, Weston Turville, Nr. Aylesbury, Bucks
Stoke Mandeville 2235

Run by severely disabled people who use Possum (electronic aid) equipment themselves and who wish to make its use known and available to others similiarly disabled. The Possum Electronic aid equipment is mouth-operated and allows a disabled person to exercise remote control over up to eleven electrical household devices Systems are also produced to operate individual items such as electric typewriters, tape recorders, dictation machines and any form of keyboard operated apparatus.

PREGNANCY ADVISORY AND MEDICAL TRUST
(P.A.M.)
64/66, Oxford Street, London W1N 9FF
01 580 4847

Assists those women who require a termination of pregnancy under the Abortion Act 1967, but who cannot obtain this on the N.H.S. and cannot afford the fees charged for a private operation.

Pre-School Playgroups Association
Alford House, Aveline Street, London SE11 5DJ

Scottish Pre-School Playgroups Association
304 Maryhill Road, Glasgow NW

The aims of the PPA are to promote the formation of playgroups (Centres provided by parents in premises approved by the Local Authority) and to press for more nursery schools and classes; to set and maintain high standards in playgroups and to increase public awareness of their value.

Preservation of the Rights of Prisoners
(PROP)
339 Finchley Road, London NW3 5HE
01 435 1215

PROP exists to try to bring about reform in the present penal system and an all-round improvement of conditions. It is a prisoners' union and full membership is open to any person who is or has been an inmate of any detention centre, remand centre, approved school, Borstal, prison or other penal establishment. Associate membership is open to all others.

Psoriasis Association
300 Wellingborough Road, Northampton NN1 4EP

Aims to increase understanding, both by patients and others, of the chronic skin disease *psoriasis* and to bring together people with this disability. Membership is open to sufferers, their relatives and anyone else interested. A newsletter is published biannually.

Psychiatric Rehabilitation Association
21a Kingsland High Street, Dalston, London E8
01 254 9753

Promotes the rehabilitation of the mentally sick, starting with preparatory work in the hospital and continuing with after-care in the community.

Queen Elizabeth's Foundation for the Disabled
Leatherhead, Surrey KT22 0BN
Oxshott 2204

Comprises four units which provide assessment, further education, vocational training, residential sheltered work, holidays and convalescence for many hundreds of disabled men and women each year.

Race Relations Board
5 Lower Belgrave Street, London SW1 0NR
01 730 6291

People who feel they have suffered unlawful discrimination on account of colour, race, ethnic or national origins, in the provision of goods, facilities and services, employment and housing, can complain to the Board, who will investigate their complaint fully.

Relaxation for Living
Dunesk, 29 Burwood Park Road, Walton-on-Thames,
Surrey KT12 5LH
Walton-on-Thames 27826

An association formed to teach people how they can help themselves to ease stress by learning to recognise quickly the build-up of tension and strain. Physical relaxation may appear easy, but it is a skill that needs to be learnt, and group classes are held to help with mental and physical relaxation. Details of classes and fees given on application.

Release
1 Elgin Avenue, London W9
01 289 1123
01 603 8654 *24-hour emergency number*

A general advice/information service to help people charged with drug offences and to deal with social, medical and legal problems caused by drugs. Specialises in advice about searches, arrests, court procedure and civil rights. On some nights lawyers are available to give free advice. Release also has a team of doctors with experience of drug users who can be consulted on any psychiatric or medical problem.

RICHMOND FELLOWSHIP
8 Addison Road, Kensington, London W14 8AL
01 603 6373/4/5

An organisation which runs halfway houses for the mentally and emotionally disturbed who are either on the way to a breakdown or have had one. People from the age of 14 can stay in the therapeutic atmosphere of the 21 houses throughout the country for varying lengths of time. The houses include some for recovering alcoholics or drug users, adolescents, etc., and referrals are made through a psychiatrist or social worker.

ROYAL ASSOCIATION IN AID OF THE DEAF AND DUMB
7/11 Armstrong Road, London, W3 7JL
01 743 6187

The Association works in London, Middlesex, Surrey, Essex and West Kent and provides special churches and social and sports clubs, with trained staff to act as interpreters and to help and advise with everyday problems. It also has specialist workers who help deaf and deaf-blind patients in psychiatric and subnormal hospitals.

ROYAL BRITISH LEGION
48/49 Pall Mall, London SW1Y 5JY
01 930 8131

ROYAL BRITISH LEGION (SCOTLAND)
23 Drumsheugh Gardens, Edinburgh EH3 7RR

An organisation which unites all men and women who have served in any of the Forces. Assistance is given with pension matters and in finding homes and employment. Financial help is offered to widows and dependants. The Legion runs a poppy factory, a Cambrian tweed factory, a British Legion Village, five country homes for the sick and aged and four convalescent homes.

Royal National Institute for the Blind
224 Great Portland Street, London W1N 6AA
01 387 5251

Promotes and organises the better education, training, employment and welfare of the blind. The R.N.I.B. runs special schools for blind children, Homes of Recovery for newly blind civilians, training schools, holiday and residential homes, and produces a wide range of educational, industrial and recreational appliances and apparatus.

Royal National Institute for the Deaf
105 Gower Street, London WC1E 6AH
01 387 8033

Acts generally to encourage the prevention and mitigation of deafness and the better treatment, education, training, employment and welfare of the deaf. The institute has six homes for the deaf, a hostel for deaf working boys, a residential training centre for maladjusted deaf youths, and a special residential school for maladjusted deaf children.

S.A.C.R.O. (Scottish Association for the Care and Resettlement of Offenders) *see* N.A.C.R.O.

Salvation Army
101 Queen Victoria Street, London EC4
01 236 5222

The Army's mission is caring, preaching, teaching, healing and saving. Amongst its multitude of welfare activities, the Salvation Army's missing-persons bureaux are perhaps best known and are remarkably successful. The Army runs Sunday schools; training colleges; music schools; homes for the aged; children's homes; centres for alcoholics and drug addicts; maternity homes for unmarried mothers; institutes for the blind; street rescue homes; approved schools; boarding schools; industrial homes; holiday homes and camps; goodwill centres; prison visits. The Army can also take action to deal with emergencies and disasters.

SAMARITANS INCORPORATED
Registered office: 17 Uxbridge Road, Slough, Bucks.
Slough 32713/4

There are at present 115 Samaritan branches in the U.K. and their sole object is to help the suicidal and despairing. A 24-hour confidential telephone service is maintained and can be used by anyone who is in despair. They will be answered by people who are unshockable and totally committed to helping by talking things out, however long it may take. (Look in the telephone book or ring directory inquiries for the number of your local branch.)

SCOTTISH ASSOCIATION FOR MENTAL HEALTH *see* MIND

SCOTTISH COUNCIL FOR THE CARE OF SPASTICS *see* SPASTICS SOCIETY

SCOTTISH COUNCIL OF SOCIAL SERVICE *see* NATIONAL COUNCIL OF SOCIAL SERVICE

SCOTTISH EPILEPSY ASSOCIATION *see* BRITISH EPILEPSY ASSOCIATION

SCOTTISH MARRIAGE GUIDANCE COUNCIL *see* NATIONAL MARRIAGE GUIDANCE COUNCIL

SCOTTISH MINORITIES GROUP
214 Clyde Street, Glasgow G1 4JZ
041 771 7600
041 334 5583

A campaigning organisation whose aim is to try to bring about a change in Scottish law relating to homosexual conduct and an end to legal and social discrimination against homosexuals. The Organisation is also able to offer help and advice to anyone with a homosexual problem. Weekly discussions and socials are held by local groups.

SCOTTISH PRE-SCHOOL PLAYGROUPS ASSOCIATION *see* PRE-SCHOOL PLAYGROUPS ASSOCIATION

SESAME
Bishop's Hall, 8 Ayres Street, London SE1 1ES
01 407 2159

Sesame offers to the mentally and physically sick and the handicapped, who are in hospitals or other centres, the opportunity for participation in drama. They arrange demonstrations (under professional direction) by mime, movement and dance groups which gradually draw their audiences into full participation. Sesame also trains occupational therapists, nurses, teachers and others working with sick and elderly people. Films suitable for teaching can be bought or hired from their office.

SHAFTESBURY SOCIETY
112 Regency Street, London SW1P 4AX
01 834 2656

Provides Christian social service to the needy or physically handicapped of all ages in thirty-three missions and youth centres in the London area. The Society runs five residential schools for crippled children, one residential centre for the young chronic sick, and two residential centres for young men suffering from muscular dystrophy. It also runs clubs and holiday centres for the physically handicapped.

SHARE COMMUNITY LIMITED
170 Kingston Road, Merton Park, London SW19 3NX
01 542 6241

Helps people to help themselves by setting up a variety of work schemes which encourage physically disabled people to meet on a friendly basis, and at the same time enjoy paid employment and responsibility to the limit of their capabilities. The schemes include printing by offset litho, pottery, toy making and a shop.

SHELTER
(National Campaign for the Homeless)
86 Strand, London WC2R 0EQ
01 836 2051

A pressure group which aims to bring to the attention of the public the plight of the homeless and the urgency of their need. Through neighbourhood action projects and advisory centres, help and advice is given to the homeless and the self-help squatting groups.

SILVER LINING APPEAL of the National Kidney Research Fund
Oakhanger Place, Nr. Bordon, Hampshire
Bordon 2021

This organisation gives help and advice to the many hundreds of suffers from renal diseases and renal failure. It also compaigns for funds and for greater supplies of donor kidneys.

SIMON COMMUNITY
49 Gansing Road, St. Leonards-on-Sea, Sussex
Hastings 6384 *must be dialled through operator*

Projects cover a multitude of problems relating to homelessness and rootlessness. Housing, both 'stop-gap' and long-term, is provided for people who, in addition to homeless, have additional problems, such as alcoholism, drug addiction or sexual deviancy, and for ex-psychiatric patients and discharged prisoners. The Community operates in a number of cities throughout the country, including Belfast.

Slimming Magazine Slimming Clubs

Slimming Magazine Limited, Burwood House, 16 Caxton Street, London SW1H 0QH
01 222 4134/8

Over 500 clubs at centres in England, Wales and Scotland provide weekly encouragement to dieters in the form of group therapy. New members complete a detailed questionnaire which is sent to the company's head office for examination by qualified dietitians. A wide range of basic diets is available – all of which have been scientifically tested and medically approved – and the most suitable is chosen for each member, with personal adjustments if necessary. Local Group Leaders, selected and trained by *Slimming Magazine*, work closely with the dietitians and nutritionists at the head office. The company also owns its own slimming hydro – Ragdale Hall in Leicestershire. Enrolment procedure and weekly details given on application.

Society for the Mutual Aid of Parents of Handicapped Children

8 Lonsdale Road, Leamington
Leamington 22807

Offers comfort and help to parents by discussion and exchange of information. Also acts as a pressure group to ensure that the needs of handicapped people are taken into account in the design and refitting of buildings and in the design of road and pedestrian schemes.

Society for the Protection of Unborn Children

47 Eaton Place, London SW1X 8DE
01 235 5268

The S.P.U.C. feels that abortion is a symptom of the failure of society and that aborting a child is often condoning bad social conditions. They aim to press for greater social justice and benefits and they have established a number of organisations to help pregnant women and girls faced with any kind of pressure to have an unwanted abortion.

Society of St. Vincent de Paul
24 George Street, London W1H 5RB
01 935 7625

A Christian, non-political society which takes an active part in works of mercy – visiting and relieving the poor; prison and hospital visiting; aiding the deaf, dumb and blind and assisting generally all those in distress and need.

Soldiers' Sailors' and Airmen's Families Association
27 Queen Anne's Gate, London SW1
01 839 4131

The objects of this Association are to provide a welfare and advisory service for the families of service and ex-service men and women; to help them to obtain benefits from all sources, both government and service, to which they may be entitled; to help ease distress with grants and to represent the cause of families in distress to the appropriate government departments where there is need to do so.

SOS Society
14 Culford Gardens, London, SW3 2SU
01 584 3717

Concerned with the establishment and maintenance of hostels for men and youths, homes for old people, and small, individual after-care hostels for mental patients.

Spare Parts Club U.K.
79 Jevington Way, London SE12

A mutual aid society for people who have undergone or require major heart surgery. Members give sympathy, understanding and encouragement to those returning to normal life after an operation, and hope to those about to have an operation. The aim of the club is also to provide financial help when necessary, not only for members in need, but also for medical research.

Spastics Society
72 Park Crescent, London W1N 4EQ
01 636 5020

Scottish Council for the Care of Spastics
22 Corstorphine Road, Edinburgh EH12 6HP
031 337 2804

Supported by 173 local groups, the Society has established 140 schools, education centres, residential homes, workshops, etc., throughout England and Wales. It has also financed a £2,000,000 research programme at Guy's Hospital, London, to discover the causes of spasticity and means of prevention.

Spinal Injuries Association
24 Nutford Place, London W1H 6AN
01 262 2641

Concerned with collecting and disseminating information on all aspects of the care of paraplegics and tetraplegics. The S.I.A. acts as a referral agency for information on equipment, benefits and help available through statutory services and voluntary agencies. It also provides information on education, further education and employment facilities and plans to produce a number of leaflets on a very wide range of subjects of interest to people suffering from spinal injuries.

Sue Ryder Foundation
Cavendish, Suffolk
Glemsford 252

Started to help survivors of concentration camps and their children, the Foundation runs three homes for physically and mentally handicapped and disabled people of different age groups.

The Association for Children with Heart Disorders
97 Mooreway, Rainhill, Liverpool L35 6PD
Prescot 2625

Primarily a pressure group to persuade the Government to release more funds to improve facilities for investigating and treating children with heart disorders. At present some children are having to wait years for heart operations which should, ideally, be carried out immediately. A Welfare Officer appointed by the Association informs parents of their civil rights, and provides services to assist needy cases.

THE BACK PAIN ASSOCIATION
Grundy House, Somerset Road, Teddington TW11 8TD

This association is trying to set up a Research Centre, founded by private donation, to find ways of solving and preventing this modern scourge. In the meantime, it is operating an information service for the medical profession.

THE BRITISH NUTRITION FOUNDATION
Alembic House, 93 Albert Embankment, London SE1 7TY
01 735 8201

Established by the food industry, the Foundation's objects are to promote education and research in nutrition and to provide authoritative information about nutrition in all its aspects. Booklets on healthy eating are available from them, including one for the elderly and one for pregnant women.

THE COMPASSIONATE FRIENDS
8 Westfield Road, Rugby, Warwickshire CV22 6AS
Rugby 5087

A group of parents who have lost a child and aim to offer friendship and understanding to other bereaved parents by helping them to come to terms with their loss.

THE CREDITON PROJECT
West Longsight, Crediton, Devon

A project which promotes vasectomy as a method of birth control for the husband in a stable marriage with a completed family, when other methods of contraception have proved unacceptable or unreliable.

THE FAMILY FUND
Joseph Rowntree Memorial Trust, Beverley House, Shipton Road, York YO3 6RB
York 29241

A Fund to help families with severely congenitally handicapped children under 16. Help is given in the form of transport assistance, holidays, clothing, laundry equipment, adaptations to houses and a practically unlimited stock of unusual aids not normally provided by Local Authorities, which include things like central heating and deep freezers, special riding saddles and toughened glass spectacles.

THE HELPING HAND ORGANISATION LIMITED
8 Strutton Ground, London SW1
01 222 6862/3

A group of 10 projects offering both residential and non-residential support to drug addicts and recovering alcoholics. The majority of referrals are from statutory or voluntary organisations, although enquiries can be made direct by the public. Most projects are in the London area but there are two in the Manchester area.

THE HOME FARM TRUST
57 Queen Square, Bristol BS1 4LF
Bristol 292060

Three houses in the country which provide home, work and security for the mentally handicapped after they leave school. Further homes are to be opened soon.

THE INSTITUTE OF SOCIAL PSYCHIATRY
115/121 Newington Causeway, London SE1 8SE
01 407 2311

An out-patient clinic (introductions preferable but not essential) for people suffering from psychiatric complaints including neurotic, psychotic and psychopathic disorders, social maladjustments (shyness, loneliness, anti-social behaviour) and family and marital disharmonies. The Clinic is staffed by experienced professionals, including consultant psychiatrists and psychotherapists.

The Link Centre for Deafened People
c/o Princess Alice Memorial Hospital, Eastbourne,
Sussex BN21 2AX
Eastbourne 22744

Aims to help to rehabilitate those who, in adult life, have to face the experience of total or severe deafness. The object of Link is to invite deaf people (with a friend or member of their family) to stay in Eastbourne in the company of those who understand their problems and have the professional ability to assist. Because of the age range, stage of adjustment and degree of deafness, each person's programme is tailor-made. Guests stay with local families or (in the case of someone with normal hearing) in a small hotel.

The National Association for Relief of Paget's Disease
413 Middleton Road, Rhodes, Middleton, Manchester M24 4QZ
061 643 1998

A fund-raising organisation to help provide equipment for research into this hereditary complaint.

The Open Door
4 Manor Brook, Blackheath, London SE3
01 852 8651

An information and contact service for those who suffer from agoraphobia (fear of open spaces). A monthly newsletter is circulated among members, through which they swap experiences and symptoms and offer advice. Members can remain anonymous, or can be put in touch with other members in the district.

The Open University
Walton Hall, Milton Keynes MK7 6AA
Milton Keynes 74066 Ext. 3722

No qualifications are needed to study with the Open University and any U.K. resident over 21 can apply. (There is also a special scheme for 18 to 21 year olds.) Students work at home, can attend one of the University's 250 study centres and are assigned a tutor-counsellor. The senior counsellor for disabled students is Geoffrey Tudor. For most students, an Open University degree takes five to six years of part-time study but some complete a degree in two or three years. Teaching is by correspondence material backed up by radio and television programmes and in their first year all students must take one of five broad-based inter-disciplinary courses: Arts, Social Sciences, Maths, Science or Technology. After that they can choose any of over 70 courses available. Fees are £25 a year with an extra £37 for a one-week summer school where applicable. Help with these costs is available from most local authorities.

The Partially-Sighted Society

Exhall Grange School, Wheelwright Lane, Coventry CV7 9HP
Coventry 87334

The Society includes among its members partially sighted people of all ages, parents of partially sighted children and many professional people who are keen to help the Society in every possible way. The aims are to promote the educational needs of all partially-sighted children and adults and to assemble and disseminate information on the help available to them. Several leaflets and booklets on specific visual handicaps are published.

The Peter Bedford Project

42/44 Aberdeen Park, Highbury, London N5

Aims, by the provision of work projects and housing, to offer single homeless and rootless people a job and a place to live. The Project helps ex-prisoners, alcoholics and ex-psychiatric patients – many of whom had been written off as unemployable – to do things to help themselves, and, by surmounting their own obstacles, to regain their self-respect and dignity.

The Phobics Society

4 Cheltenham Road, Chorlton-cum-Hardy, Manchester M21 1QN
Chorlton-cum-Hardy 1937

There are an estimated 4,000,000 phobics (anxiety-state sufferers) in the British Isles. The Phobics Society has branches established or starting in various parts of the country (including Northern Ireland) and is planning to open a centre in Manchester where there will be social and therapeutic activities designed to relieve tensions. The aims of the Society are to promote medical and other therapies and research into the causes and cure of phobias, to assist in rehabilitation and to provide after-care. Advice will be given by post if s.a.e. is sent.

THE RENAL SOCIETY
64 South Hill Park, London NW3

Gives encouragement to kidney patients, especially those who have to cope with a stringent diet. The Society was established to enable people to exchange views and recipes; to publish information about any new protein-free and salt-free products that come on the market; to give information concerning possible financial help in certain cases. Contacts are made through a bi-monthly Newsletter which includes a register of members who may wish to contact each other.

THE RESPONAUT
39 Essex Street, Newbury, Berks

The magazine *Responaut* disseminates information. Its purpose is to restore natural liberties to disabled people by showing the strengths and weaknesses of welfare services, statutory, voluntary and commercial, and to discuss equipment and ideas. Its contributors and readers cover a wide spectrum.

THE SCHIZOPHRENIA FELLOWSHIP OF GREAT BRITAIN
Victoria Road, Surbiton, Surrey
01 390 3651/2

A recently formed national Association which aims to spread information and understanding of the illness. They believe that correct food helps to alleviate the illness and plan to urge the Government to spend more money on research into the possible physical and biochemical causes of schizophrenia.

The Scout Association
25 Buckingham Palace Road, London SW1W 0PY
01 834 6005

The Scout Movement's policy is to encourage the integration of handicapped boys into normal society and particularly in connection with Scouting. Wherever possible, Scouts with a handicap are encouraged to belong to an ordinary Group. Obviously, handicapped children may find some of the Scout programme impossible to accomplish and for them there are Extension Activities which are more suitable, absorbing, worth while and enjoyable for boys who are physically or mentally handicapped. The home-bound boy may also participate through membership of a local Group.

The Society of Skin Camouflage
Doreen Savage Trust, Balhepburn, Rhynd, Perth, Scotland
Perth 23519

The aims of this Society are to establish, within the framework of the National Health Service, a Skin Camouflage Structure and Training programme as an essential part of the emotional rehabilitation of patients with major or minor facial or body skin defects. Some Camouflage Clinics are in operation in hospitals under the N.H.S., and the procedure for obtaining help from them is to ask your doctor for a referral to the Consultant Dermatologist or Consultant Plastic Surgeon at one of these hospitals. A magazine, *Talk about Camouflage,* is published and further information can be obtained by telephoning or writing to the Trust, enclosing a s.a.e.

The St. Mungo Community Trust
39/42 Battersea High Street, London SW11 3JF
01 223 4444

Best known for the 'soup run', St. Mungo's – a non-religious organisation – feeds several hundred down-and-outs in Central London between midnight and 4.30 a.m. This meal of soup and bread is often the only meal of the day for people living on the streets, but, most important, the soup run provides an opportunity for contact for people who are often suspicious, isolated, withdrawn and reticent. Helpers are needed all the time. St. Mungo's is also deeply involved in providing accommodation and support for homeless men in London and in a number of long-term care and rehabilitation projects. They run a shop in which some of the men work and 'Com-care', a community transport service.

THE THISTLE FOUNDATION
22 Charlotte Square, Edinburgh EH2 4DF
031 225 7282/8484

The Foundation administers a 'village' of 103 houses and a hostel which accommodate single and married disabled people and their families. Each house is linked by a covered way to a central clinic, physiotherapy and occupational therapy departments, gymnasium swimming pool and recreation hall. The Foundation is responsible for the upkeep of the houses but residents are expected to furnish them and pay for their own living expenses.

TOC H
Forest Close, Wendover, Bucks
Wendover 3256

A movement open to all, with more than 1400 branches in the U.K. It exists so that men and women may test the truth of the Christian faith and its relevance to everyday life. It asks that they involve themselves unreservedly in the community and so find that life holds meaning and purpose for all who see the needs of others as their own. In many cities residential houses known as 'Marks' provide bases for social activity and constructive community relations.

TOY LIBRARIES ASSOCIATION FOR HANDICAPPED CHILDREN
Toynbee Hall, 28 Commercial Street, London E1 6LS
01 247 1497

Centres which are equipped for lending the best, and often specially adapted, toys to handicapped children which stimulate their imagination, teach them skills and help them to become more socially involved. The 70 operating libraries also provide a local meeting place for parents, children and professional people. A number of publications are available including one which gives do-it-yourself instructions on making noisy, rewarding, play material for a child who has rejected all toy shop toys.

U & I Club
22 Gerrard Road, Islington, London N1 8AY

Gives advice to members on all aspects of urinary infection. A bi-monthly magazine is published, containing case histories, ideas and remedies, with particular reference to cystitis.

United Kingdom Immigrants' Advisory Service
St. George's Churchyard, 38 Bloomsbury Way, London WC1A 2SA

Advises Commonwealth citizens and aliens who are in difficulties with immigration control, and, where necessary, assists them in presenting their case to the Home Office and the appellate authorities.

Wales Council for the Disabled
(In association with the Council of Social Service for Wales)
2 Cathedral Road, Cardiff CF1 9XR
Cardiff 21456/8

Brings together the many organisations working for the disabled in Wales: disabled action groups, voluntary welfare organisations, professional bodies and statutory authorities. Information on holidays, sports, education, day and residential care, employment and personal income is available to the public, together with information and guidance on specific disablements.

Weight Watchers
1 Thames Street, Windsor, Berkshire SL4 1SW
Windsor 69131

Started in America when a fifteen-stone woman found it difficult to discuss her weight problem with a slim specialist. Now a national institution in Britain. Newcomers to classes are measured to check what their weight should be and their eating habits are appraised. Members then weigh in regularly: loss is applauded and gain discussed. Ninety-three per cent of members lose weight and their maintenance of weight loss is equally impressive.

Wider Horizons
Crag House, Woodland Road, Windermere,
Cumbria LA23 2AN

Promotes wider interests among handicapped and housebound people, primarily by the publication of a bi-monthly magazine written by handicapped members. All contacts are made by correspondence and a Modern Aids Fund has been set up which will assist disabled members to obtain equipment such as typewriters and tape recorders when these are not available from other sources.

Winged Fellowship Trust
79/80 Petty France, London SW1H 9HB
01 222 3589

Provides a two-week holiday for as many severely handicapped people as possible and so gives the families of the disabled a break. The Trust also provides a challenging voluntary service for people of all ages. The volunteers live with the disabled guests for two weeks and become their 'arms and legs', their companions and friends.

Wingfield Trust
24 Station Road, Epping
Epping 3229

Helps physically handicapped children and young people to overcome their disabilities through music and other activities. There are eight Wingfield Music Clubs in London which meet one evening a week for two hours. Every newcomer is taught the recorder first. While he is learning this, teachers study him to see which instrument best suits his disability. There are also cycle clubs which supply specially adapted machines, and a number of other aids to help propulsion have been developed by the Trust.

Women's Aid
396 Chiswick High Road, London W4

Started as a local centre for the women of Chiswick, aimed at providing an informal meeting place where problems of housing, children, contraception, abortion, household finances and so on could be discussed and resolved. The organisation has now become a national centre dealing with the major social problem of the battered woman. As well as helping by sheltering, advising and caring for women who have been persistently beaten by their husbands, Women's Aid cares for the children, often helping to clothe them. There is no 'average' length of stay at the centre. Some cases are dealt with speedily with the help of solicitors, doctors and social workers whom the group have recruited to assist. More serious cases remain in almost permanent residence until alternative accommodation can be found for them.

Women's League of Health and Beauty
Beamont Cottage, Ditton Close, Thames Ditton, Surrey
01 398 3719

The League exists to improve the standard of health and the health consciousness of women throughout the U.K. Health exercise and movement classes are held and displays and rallies are attended by members from all parts of Britain. Part-time training courses are also available for girls who wish to take up League teaching as a career.

Women's Liberation Workshop
38 Earlham Street, London WC2
01 836 6081

A radical feminist organisation which believes that women in our society are oppressed and commercially exploited. The Workshop is composed of small groups which meet weekly. Each group is autonomous and acts as a watchdog and pressure group to try to re-define woman's role in society and broaden her horizons, and helps, in a practical sense, by making literature and discussion freely available.

Women's National Cancer Control Campaign
9 King Street, London, WC2E 8HN
01 836 9901

Help and advice is given about the preventive side of cervical and breast cancer screening. A comprehensive range of leaflets is issued, including one in six languages for the immigrant population. There is a daily 'answer service' for women who have problems on these subjects. Leaflets giving advice to women who are to undergo a breast operation and on after-care will soon be available.

W.R.V.S.
(Women's Royal Voluntary Service)
17 Old Park Lane, London W1Y 4AJ
01 499 6040

Their Good Companions Scheme helps handicapped and aged people who are finding it increasingly difficult to run their homes without assistance. Among duties undertaken by volunteers are escorting patients to hospital out-patients departments or to the opticians, cleaning windows, ironing, shopping, taking clothes to the laundry and the thousand and one other daily and emergency household tasks which occur in the running of a home.

Section 3

Where to get more information

This section lists a selection of books and pamphlets about health and social welfare, classified by subject. These books should be available through your local library and many are currently on sale. Where possible we have given dates of publication and current prices but these are obviously subject to revision. If your local bookshop will not accept an order for any of these books, you may still be able to order the book by post from W. G. Foyle Ltd., 119 Charing Cross Road, London WC2.

ABORTION

Abortion Law Reformed — 1971 — £3·25
by K. Hindell and M. Simms
Peter Owen

Abortion Now — 20p
Abortion Law Reform Association

Abortion: The Personal Dilemma — 1972 — £1·25
by R. F. Gardner
Paternoster Press

A Guide to the Abortion Act 1967 — 20p
Abortion Law Reform Association

The New Abortion Law: How it affects you (leaflet) — 2½p
Abortion Law Reform Association

ADDICTION

Alcohol

About the Illness Alcoholism — 1972 — 20p
by W. Kenyon
National Council on Alcoholism

Alcohol and Drug Dependence: treatment and rehabilitation — 1972 — £1·50
by W. P. James et al.
King Edwards's Hospital Fund

The Alcoholic and the Help He Needs — 1972 — £3·25
by M. Glatt
Priory Press 2nd edition

Alcoholism — 1966 — £1·50
by N. Kessel and H. Walton — Penguin 30p
MacGibbon and Kee

Facilities for the Treatment of Alcoholism — 1973 — Gratis
(Directory of organisations offering help to alcoholics)
Medical Council on Alcoholism

DRUGS

Addicts, Drugs and Alcohol Re-examined — 1973 — £2·25
by J. Willis
Pitman Publishing Co.

The Adolescent Gap: research findings on drug-using and non-drug-using teens — 1972 — £3·15
by E. M. Scott

Behind the Drug Scene — 15p
by M. Schofield
British Medical Association Family Doctor Booklet

Drug Dependence — 1967 — 12½p
by A. J. Wood
Bristol Corporation and Bristol Council of Social Service

Drug Dependence: a study for nurses and social workers — (1969) £1·10; 1970 55p paperback
by J. H. Willis
Faber and Faber

Body and Drug — 1973 — £2·75
edited by M. Jefferies
Sociopack Publication

Drugs and Human Behaviour *by* G. Claridge Pelican	1972	40p
Drug scene in Great Britain: Journey into Loneliness *by* M. Glatt et al. Edward Arnold	1967	80p
Drugs, Alcohol and Tobacco in Britain *by* J. Zacune and C. Hensman W. Heinemann Medical Books	1972	£4·00
Drugs for Young People: their use and misuse *by* K. Leech and B. Jordan Religious Education Press	(1967) 1970	60p
Drugs from A–Z: a dictionary *by* R. R. Lingeman A. Lane	1969	£3·35 £2·50
Drugs Misuse and the Law *by* S. Bradshaw Macmillan	1972	95p
Drugs: the parent's dilemma *by* A. R. K. Mitchell Priory Press Ltd. 4th edition	1973	80p
Misuse of Drugs Act H.M.S.O. (Repeals Drugs (Prevention of Misuse Act) 1967 and Dangerous Drugs Act, 1965 and 1967)	1971	30p
The New Families: youth communes and the politics of drugs *by* R. V. Speck et al. Tavistock Publications	1972	£2·50
Pot or Not: a plain guide to drug dependence *by* A. J. Wood British Medical Association Family Doctor Booklet	1969	15p

Where on Drugs *edited by* B. McAlhone Advisory Centre for Education, Cambridge	1970	35p
The Willing Victim: a parents' guide to drug abuse *by* C. Birdwood Secker and Warburg	1969	£2·10
Young Outsiders: a study of alternative communities *by* R. Mills Routledge and Kegan Paul	1973	£3·00

TOBACCO

Facts about Smoking and Young People Chest and Heart Association	1971	
Smoking and Health Now: a report and summary on smoking and its effect on health *by* The Royal College of Physicians Pitman Publishing Co.	1971	50p
Smoking, Lung Cancer and You *by* R. M. McCurdy Linden	1972	60p
When and How to Stop Smoking *by* E. Chesser Jarrolds	1963	10s 6d o.p.

AGED

REJUVENATION

Age and Vitality: commonsense ways of adding life to your years *by* I. Gore G. Allen and Unwin	1973	£2·25
Be Fit at 40 *by* D. Featherston Thorsons	1965	75p

Health for Old Age *edited by* E. Rudinger Consumers Association	1973	75p
How Not to Die Young *by* J. Gomez G. Allen and Unwin	1973	£2·50
Live Long and Stay Young *by* E. Trimmer G. Allen and Unwin	1965	75p
Ageing *by* A. Comfort Routledge *replaces*	[1965]	£2·50
Process of Ageing *by* A. Comfort Weidenfeld and Nicolson	1965	
Rejuvenation *by* E. Trimmer Robert Hale Ltd.	1967	£1·25
Sixty Plus *by* J. Maddison and K. Hastrop British Medical Association Family Doctor Booklet	1970	15p
An Approach to Old Age and its Problems *by* M. N. Hill Oliver and Boyd	1961	75p o.p.
The Care of the Aged *by* D. Hyams Priory Press Ltd.	1972	£2·25 and 80p
Caring for the Elderly *by* G. Francis W. Heinemann Medical Books	1973	90p
Good Neighbours National Old People's Welfare Council	1972	7p

Helping the Elderly: personal hints with advice to relatives and friends *by* F. L. Willington and G. P. Jones National Council for the Elderly in Wales and Council for the Social Services in Wales and Monmouthshire	1972	
Human Relations in Old Age *by* T. N. Rudd Faber and Faber (A handbook for health visitors, social workers and others)	(1967) 1969	£1·10
New Housing for the Elderly: a study of housing schemes for the elderly provided by the Hanover Housing Association *by* D. Page and T. Muir Bedford Square Press for the National Corporation for the Care of Old People	1971	75p

RETIREMENT

The Executive and the Seventies – Men Only *by* B. Williamson Lloyd – Luke	1973	£1·25
Future Perfect: retirement planning and management *by* E. Samson Kimpton	1972	£1·75
A Guide to Activities for Older People *by* W. M. Gwyneth Elek Books	1970	12s 6d o.p.
Money Guide: notes for the retired on pensions. taxes, allowances, concessions, savings *by* S. Coghill Age Concern National Old People's Welfare Council	1973	20p
A Practical Guide to Retirement *by* G. St. John Murray Epworth Press	1970	35p

Pre-retirement and Retirement *by* J. P. McErlean (Available from author at 24 Graeme Road, Enfield, EN1 3U8	1973	50p
Retirement a Pleasure: or out but not down *by* H. Yoxall Elm Tree Books; Hamish Hamilton	1971	£1·60
Rights of Old People National Secular Society	1972	15p
Work, Age and Leisure: causes and consequence of the shortened working life *by* F. le Gros Clark Michael Joseph	1966	£1·50
Your Rights *by* P. Hewitt Age Concern National Old People's Welfare Council	1973	10p

ALLERGIES

ASTHMA, HAYFEVER, FOOD

Allergies *by* D. B. Macaulay Priory Press Ltd.	1973	£2·50
Allergies, Asthma, Hay Fever, Dermatitis, Migraine, et al. *by* F. E. Graham–Bonnalie David and Charles	1970	£1·25
Asthma and Hay Fever and Other Allergic Disorders, for Victims and their Families *by* O. Swineford Thomas (Springfield, U.S.A.)	1973	$10·75
Asthma: a guide for patients *by* K. M. Hume Chest and Heart Association	1970	80p

Asthma and How to Live With It — 15p
by W. Benson
British Medical Association Family Doctor

Asthma and Other Allergies: an explanation for the layman — 1970 — $1·00
by E. Phillipp
Reed (New Zealand)

Food Allergies and the Allergic Patient — 1973 — £1·80
by E. L. Taube
Thomas (Springfield, U.S.A.)

A Parent's Guide to Children's Allergies — 1972 — $8·00 and $3·95 paperback
by E. Somekh
Thomas (Springfield, U.S.A.)

Understanding Allergies — 1973 — $3·95
by J. W. Gerrard
Thomas (Springfield, U.S.A.)

You and Your Allergy — 1971 — 15p
by D. B. Macaulay
British Medical Association Family Doctor Booklet

Your Allergic Child — 1970 — 60p
by H. Hirschfield
Arc Books (U.S.A. (1964))

BACKACHE

The Alexander Principle — 1973 — £3·00
by W. Barlow
Gollancz

Backache in Women — 1966 — £1·20
by E. Schlayer-Saunders
John Wright. 2nd edition

Backache, Stress and Tension: their cause prevention and treatment — 1966 — £1·50
by H. Krauss
G. Allen and Unwin

Manual of Osteopathic Practice *by* A. Stoddard Hutchinson Medical Publications	1969	£3·50
Relief Without Drugs: self management and tension *by* A. Meares Collins/Fontana		30p
Remedial Exercise for Postural Defects: for use in the home and school *compiled by* L. S. Rolleston John Wright	1955	20p
Slipped Disc *by* J. Cyriax Gower Press	1970	£2·10
So You Know About Poise and Relaxation *by* N. Capener British Medical Association Family Doctor Booklet	1969	15p
You are as Young as Your Spine *by* E. Hearn W. Heinemann Medical Books (slipped discs, backache, rheumatism, sciatica)	1967	90p

BEREAVEMENT

Begin Again: a book for women alone *by* M. Torrie Dent	1970	£1·40
Bereavement: studies of grief in adult life *by* C. Murray Parkes Tavistock Publications	1972	£3·00
Grief and How to Live with It *by* S. Morris G. Allen and Unwin	1971	£1·50
Widowed *by* D. P. Jepp Mayhew McCrimmon	1973	50p

BLOOD GROUPS

Blood Groups in Man — new edition due 1974 — £10·00 approx
by R. R. Race and R. Sanger
Blackwell 5th edition

What Rhesus Negative Means — 15p
by R. A. Zeitlin
British Medical Association Family Doctor Booklet

BLOOD PRESSURE

How To Live With Your Blood Pressure — 1956 — 8s 6d o.p.
by B. Beatty
British Medical Association Family Doctor Booklet

Hypertension: causes, consequences and management — 1972 — £1·75
by Sir G. Pickering
Churchill Livingstone

The Silent Disease: Hypertension — 1973 — £2·95
by L. Galton
Nelson (Crown N.Y.)

You and Your Blood Pressure — 1971 — 15p
by H. Williams
British Medical Association Family Doctor Booklet

Your Blood Pressure and How To Live With It — 1957 — 75p
by W. A. Brams
Staples

CANCER

Cancer and Common Sense — 1957 — 10s 6d o.p.
by G. Crile
Hale

Cancer: the significance of delay *by* R. Sutherland Butterworths	1960	£1·50
Cancer If Curable, Why Not Cured? *by* J. S. Mitchell Heffer	1971	£2·00
Cancer and You *by* H. C. Lynch Thomas (Springfield, U.S.A.)	1971	$7·43
Conquest of Cancer *by* J. Wilkinson Hart-Davis, MacGibbon	1973	£3·50
Truth About Cancer *by* M. H. Kirwin British Medical Association Family Doctor Booklet	1969	15p
What We Know About Cancer *by* R. J. C. Harris G. Allen and Unwin	1970	£3·25 and £1·75

PERSONAL NARRATIVES

Atoms at Tea Time: the story of a cure *by* P. Paoli Deutsch	1968	£1·05
A Journey *by* D. Gault Chatto and Windus	1968	75p
Living with a Man who is Dying *by* J. Evans Blond	1971	£1·50
A Time to Heal *by* P. Newton-Fenbow Souvenir Press (Dr. J. Issels treatment methods)	1971	£1·75

CHEST DISEASES

Bronchitis and Tuberculosis

The Breath of Life *by* H. Day Thorsons (correct breathing)	1965	£1·00
The Chest in Health and Disease *by* K. P. Goldman Chest and Heart Association Health Horizon	1970	90p
The Chesty Child Chest and Heart Association Health Horizon	1965	30p
Conquest of Tuberculosis *by* S. A. Waksman Robert Hales Ltd.	1965	£1·50 o.p.
For Those who Live and Breathe: with emphysema and chronic bronchitis *by* L. Petty and L. M. Nett Thomas (Springfield, U.S.A.) 2nd edition	1972	£2·83
How Not To Get Chronic Bronchitis *by* J. C. Scadding British Medical Association Family Doctor Booklet	1969	15p
Living with Chronic Bronchitis Burroughs Wellcome	1971	o.p.
New Life Through Breathing *by* K. Knowles *edited by* B. Morgan G. Allen and Unwin	1966	£1·25
Requiem for a Great Killer *by* H. Williams Chest and Heart Association Health Horizon	1973	£1·50
Tuberculosis *by* S. Shaw Duckworth	1955	8s 6d o.p.
Understanding Bronchitis and Asthma *by* R. Kemp Tavistock Publications	1963	87½p

What You Can Do About Your Breathing National Tuberculosis Association	1967	o.p.

CHILD HEALTH

Babies and Young Children *by* R. and S. Illingworth Churchill Livingston (Recommended for expectant mothers and those bringing up young children)	1973	£2·50
Baby's First Days *by* J. W. Partridge Priory Press Ltd.	1973	£2·50
Child Care and Management: from birth to adolescence *by* P. Edge Faber and Faber 3rd edition	1971	£2·25 and 75p
Common Ailments in Babies *by* R. S. Illingworth British Medical Association Family Doctor Booklet		15p
Common Ailments in Toddlers *by* R. S. Illingworth British Medical Association Family Doctor Booklet		15p
Common Sense About Babies and Children *by* H. Jolly Times Newspapers	1973	40p
How Not To Kill Your Children *by* a Family Doctor G. Allen and Unwin	1968	£1·75
Growth Through Play: the first two years *by* B. Tudor Hart National Society of Children's Nurseries (available from One Parent Families)		12½p

Infectious Diseases of Childhood *by* T. Anderson British Medical Association Family Doctor Booklet		15p
The Know-How of Infant Care *by* S. Close J. Wright 2nd edition	1972	40p
The Know-How of Infant Feeding *by* S. Close J. Wright 3rd edition	1973	40p
A Pictorial Guide to Common Childhood Illness *by* G. Vaughan Arcade Publishing	1971	£2·00
Practical Parenthood *by* G. and R. Gordon Mayflower	1969	25p
Sudden and Unexpected Deaths in Infancy *edited by* F. Camps and R. G. Carpenter J. Wright (cot deaths)	1972	£2·00
Your Children's Health *by* M. Manning Elm Tree Books; Hamish Hamilton	1973	£2·10
Your Wonderful Baby: a practical approach to baby and child care *by* W. J. Potts G. Allen and Unwin	1968	£1·75 o.p.

HANDICAPPED

Aids for the Handicapped *by* N. D. B. Elwes Spastics Society	1973	50p
Autistic Children: innocents at risk National Society for Autistic Children	1968	10p

Autistic Children: a guide for parents *by* L. Wing Constable and Co.	1971	£2·00
Behaviour Problems Amongst Children with Cerebral Palsy *by* M. Oswin J. Wright	1967	80p
Cerebral Palsy and the Young Child *by* S. M. Blencowe Churchill Livingstone	1969	£1·50
Challenge of Spina Bifida *by* A. Field W. Heinemann Medical Books	1970	40p
Child With Cerebral Palsy: social, emotional and educational adjustment: an annotated bibliography *by* D. Pilling National Foundation for Educational Research	1973	
Children with Down's Syndrome *by* D. W. Smith and A. A. Wilson Saunders (Philadelphia, U.S.A.)	1973	
Developmental Handicap in Babies and Young Children: a guide for parents *by* D. L. Brown Thomas (Springfield, U.S.A.)	1972	$5·75
Directory of Voluntary Organisations Concerned with Children *edited by* M. L. K. Pringle et al. Longmans for National Bureau of Co-operation in Child Care	1969	£3·50
Dsylexia *by* T. S. Hepworth Angus and Robertson	1971	£1·75
Dyslexia and the Individual *by* P. Meredith Elm Tree Books; Hamish Hamilton	1972	£2·35

Dyslexia: a guide for teachers and parents *by* M. Newton University of Aston in Birmingham	1971	5p
Facilities Available for Autistic Children National Society for Autistic Children	1970	20p
Handbook for Parents of a Handicapped Child *by* J. Stone and F. Taylor Case Publications	1972	15p
Handicap: a study of physically handicapped children and their families *by* J. K. McMichael Staples Press	1971	£2·75
Handicapped Child: educational and psychological guide for the organically handicapped *by* A. H. Bowley and L. Gardner Churchill Livingstone 3rd edition	1972	£1·50
Handicapped Child: a research review; pts. I and II *edited by* R. Dinnage Longman for National Children's Bureau	1970 pt. I 1972 pt.II	£2·75 £3·53
Handling the Young Cerebral Palsied Child at Home *by* N. R. Finnie W. Heinemann Medical Books Ltd. (1968)	1971	£1·00
Improving Mongol Babies and Introducing Them to School *by* R. Brinkworth and J. Collins National Society for Mentally Handicapped Children (Belfast)	1973	50p
Life With a Mentally Sick Child *by* P. Lacey Pergamon	1969	£1·25 and 75p
Mental Retardation *by* B. Kirman Pergamon	1968	40p

Mentally Handicapped Child *by* B. Kirman Nelson	1972	£2·95
Mentally Handicapped Child Under Five *by* C. Dybwad National Society for Mentally Handicapped Children	1973	15p
On Helping the Dyslexic Child *by* T. R. Miles Methuen Educational	1970	£1·20
Play Activities for the Retarded Child *by* B. W. Carlson and R. R. Ginglend Baillière Tindall	1962	£2·50
Practical Help for Parents of Retarded Children: some questions and answers *by* A. M. Clarke and A. D. B. Clarke Hull Society for Mentally Handicapped Children	1969	15p
Slant Eyed Angel: with a note on Down's syndrome *by* J. Van Der Hoeven Colin Smythe	1968	£1·50 £1·05
The Spastic Schoolchild and the Outside World *by* J. Loring and A. Mason W. Heinemann and the Spastics Society	1966	75p
They Say My Child is Backward: a guide for parents and educationalists *by* C. H. Jackson National Society for Mentally Handicapped Children	1970	25p
Toys and Games for Educationally Handicapped Children *by* C. Abuist and J. L. Shulman Thomas (Springfield, U.S.A.)		$9·50

CHILD PSYCHOLOGY

Basic Child Psychiatry *by* P. Barker Staples	1971	£2·75 and £1·50
Born to Fail *by* P. Wedge and H. Prosser Arrow Books	1973	30p
Child Care and Management: from birth to adolescence *by* P. Edge Faber and Faber 3rd edition	1971	£2·25 and 75p
The Child Under Stress *by* E. Oakeshott Priory Press Ltd.	1973	80p
Children Under Stress *by* S. Woolff Pelican	1973	50p
Understanding Your Child *by* W. de Kok British Medical Association Family Doctor Booklet		15p
Your Child is a Person: a psychological approach to parenthood without guilt *by* C. Chess, A. Thomas and H. G. Birch Davies	1965	£1·05 o.p.

CHILD WELFARE

ADOPTION AND FOSTERING

Adopting a Child: a brief guide to prospective adopters Association of British Adoption Agencies	1972	15p
Adoption in Brief: research and other literature in the U.S., Canada and Great Britain 1966–1972: an annotated bibliography *by* A. A. Jack National Foundation for Educational Research	1973	£1·70

Adoption: Facts and Fallacies *by* M. L. K. Pringle Longman	1967	£1·10
Children Apart: problems of early separation from parents *by* P. Rowlands Dent	1973	£2·50
The Community's Children: long term substitute care: a guide for the intelligent layman *edited by* J. Parfit Longmans for National Bureau of Co-operation in Child Care	1967	80p
Foster Home Care: facts and fallacies *by* M. L. K. Pringle and R. Dinnage Longmans	1967	£1·85
Growing Up Adopted *by* J. Seglow, M. L. K. Pringle and P. Welch National Foundation for Educational Research	1972	£2·20
How To Adopt *by* E. Rudinger Consumers Association 3rd edition	1975	85p

DIABETES

Diabetes Explained *by* A. Bloom Medical and Technical Publishing Co. Ltd.	1971	£1·90
The Diabetic ABC: a practical guide for patients and nurses by R. D. Lawrence H. K. Lewis	1967	35p o.p.
The Diabetic at Work and Play *by* B. R. Boshell Thomas (Springfield, U.S.A.)	1971	£3·93
The Diabetic Manual for Doctor and Patient *by* E. P. Joslin Henry Kimpton (Lea and Febiger, U.S.A.)	1959	£1·70

Handbook for the Young Diabetic *by* A. E. Fischer and D. L. Horstmann Intercontinental Medical Book Corporation	1972	£2·15
Life with Diabetes *by* A. Bloom British Medical Association Family Doctor Booklet	1972	15p
Notes for Diabetics: diets and instructions given to patients attending University College Hospital H. K. Lewis	1971	20p
Notes for the Guidance of Parents of Diabetic Children *by* J. N. Farquar Churchill Livingstone	1970	25p
Your Child has Diabetes: a guide to parents and their children who have diabetes *by* J. M. Court W. Heinemann Medical Books Ltd.	1972	£1·90

RECIPES

Cooking for the Wayward Diabetic *by* L. MacLeod Faber and Faber 2nd edition	1971	£1·25
Diet Without Tears Cookery Book *by* I. H. Rogers H. K. Lewis	1973	65p
Gourmet Recipes for Diabetics *by* D. T. Revell Thomas (Springfield, U.S.A.)	1971	£4·28
List of Carbohydrates and Calorie Contents of Alcoholic Drinks British Diabetic Association	1971	

DIGESTIVE SYSTEM

Digestive System *by* R. J. Ryall Penguin Books	1973	90p

Making Friends With Your Ulcer British Medical Association Family Doctor Booklet		15p
Peptic Ulcer: a new approach to its causation, prevention, and arrest, based on human evolution *by* T. L. Cleave J. Wright	1962	£1·50
Understanding Duodenal Ulcer *by* R. Kemp Tavistock Publications	1964	17s 6d o.p.
You and Your Guts *by* E. Hawkins British Medical Association Family Doctor Booklet	1971	15p

DISABLED

AIDS

An ABC of Services and General Information for the Disabled *by* B. MacMorland Disablement Income Group		10p
Aids for the Handicapped Spastic Society	1973	50p
Catalogue of Aids for the Disabled British Red Cross Society		20p
Early Days: you and your new baby Disabled Living Foundation		£1·25
Electric Aids for Disabled People Electricity Council Marketing Department or Local Electricity Board Showrooms	1974	Gratis
A Guide to Disposable Incontinence Underpads Disabled Living Foundation		15p
A Guide to Societies and Organisations which offer Advice and Information to the Mentally and Physically Handicapped Patient's Association	1973	10p

Gas Aids the Disabled — Gratis
British Gas Corporation or Local Gas Board
Showrooms

Help Yourselves: a handbook for hemiplagics and their families
by Peggy Jay
Butterworth

Incontinence Project: references to appliances and equipment for incontinence: a select bibliography — 1971 — 50p
Disabled Living Foundation

Incontinence: some problems, suggestions and conclusions — 1970 — 80p
by L. Elphick
Disabled Living Foundation

Orthopaedic Appliances — 1972 — £2·95 and £1·45
by B. H. Day
Faber and Faber

CLOTHING

Catalogue of Garments for the Handicapped and Disabled — 1972 2 v. £5·50; Supplement 1973 £2·50
by J. Lord
King Edward's Fund for the Shirley Institute, Manchester

Clothes Sense for Handicapped Adults of all ages — £1·50
Disabled Living Foundation

Clothing Fastenings for the Handicapped and Disabled — 37½p
Disabled Living Foundation

Clothing for the Handicapped Child — 1972 — £1·20
by G. Forbes
Disabled Living Foundation

Clothing for Wheelchair Users — 20p
Disabled Living Foundation

Dressmaking for the Disabled Disabled Living Foundation		23p
Footwear for Problem Feet *by* M. D. England Disabled Living Foundation	1973	£1·25
Information Sheets on – Corsets, Foundation Garments, Stockings and Suspenders Clothing and Dressmaking for People with Stiff Hips Clothing and Incontinence Protective Garments Disabled Living Foundation		 8p 8p 8p 15p
Sewing Notes: advice on how to adapt existing clothing Disabled Living Foundation		50p
Materials and Clothing in Health and Disease *by* E. T. Renbourn H. K. Lewis	1972	£9·50
A Survey of Problems of Clothing for the Sick and Disabled Disabled Living Foundation		53p

HOME

Cleaning Equipment Disabled Living Foundation		45p
The Disabled User: vacuum cleaners Research Institute for Consumer Affairs Comparative Test Report No. 10 National Fund for Research into Crippling Diseases (covers 12 models)	1971	30p
Handicapped Child and His Home *by* M. O. Sheridan National Children's Home Sales Division	1973	50p
Home Management National Fund for Research into Crippling Diseases Guide		£1·05

An Introduction to Domestic Design for the Disabled — 63p
Disabled Living Foundation

Laundry Equipment — 30p
Disabled Living Foundation

Lists of Kitchen Equipment — 29p
Disabled Living Foundation

Living with a Handicap — 1973 — £2·95
by P. Nicholls
Priory Press

Needs of the Disabled: illustrations of furniture and equipment, storage space for clothing — 5p
Cutlery — 3p

A Pilot Study of Disabled Housewives and their Kitchens — £1·50
Disabled Living Foundation

GARDENING

Easy Path to Gardening — £1·25
Diabled Living Foundation and Reader's Digest

Set of Papers on Gardening for the Disabled: advice on tools, plants, raised flower beds — 20p
Disabled Living Foundation

Gardening for the Disabled: illustrated articles reprinted from Medical and Biological Illustration — 10p
Disabled Living Foundation

WELFARE

Access to Public Conveniences: a handbook for the disabled person — 1973 — 20p
Central Council for the Disabled

Access to University and Polytechnic Buildings: a handbook for disabled students — 1972 — 20p
Central Council for the Disabled

Communication £1·05
National Fund for Research into Crippling Diseases Guide

Disabled Students in Higher Education £1·50
by National Innovations Centre
Research Publications Services (Victoria Hall, E. Greenwich)

Handicapped School Leavers: their future education, training and employment 1973 £1·00
by L. Tuckey, J. Parfit and B. Tuckey
National Foundation for Educational Research

Help for Handicapped People 1972
Department of Health and Social Security *and* Welsh Office
(main benefits and services available)

Holidays for the Physically Handicapped 1974 40p
Central Council for the Disabled

London for the Disabled: a guide to physical features and hazards of London shops, hotels and restaurants etc. 1973 50p
Disabled Living Foundation

Music and the Physically Handicapped 1969 25p
Disabled Living Foundation

Sport and Physical Recreation for the Disabled 50p
Disabled Living Foundation

Who Looks After You at Heathrow Airport?
(Available from Central Council for Disabled; Disabled Living Foundation, 3p and S.A.E.; or British Airport Authority Information Desk)

EPILEPSY

About Epilepsy 1973 £3·45 and £1·25
by D. Scott
Duckworth 2nd edition

The Child with Convulsions: a guide for parents, educators and medical personnel | 1972 | £4·00
by H. W. Beard
Grune and Stratton

Epilepsy | 1954 | 8s 6d
by L. Fairfield | | o.p.
Duckworth's Modern Health Series

Epilepsy and Other Chronic and Convulsive Diseases: their causes, symptoms and treatment | 1964 | £1·25 (standard text book)
by W. R. Gowers
Dover Publications (N.Y., U.S.A.)

Epilepsy and Fits | | 15p
by D. Pond and E. M. Johnson
British Medical Association Family Doctor Booklet

EYES

About Your Eyes | | 15p
British Medical Association Family Doctor Booklet

Incidence and Causes of Blindness in England and Wales 1963–1968: plus appendix on social services available for incipient blindness | 1972 | 52½p
by A. Sorsby
Department of Health and Social Security. Reports on Public Health and Medical Subjects No. 128
H.M.S.O.

Lighting and Seeing: on colour vision, artificial lighting | 1969 | £1·75
by R. G. Hopkinson
W. Heineman Medical

Preservation of Eyesight | 1958 | 70p
edited by A. S. Macnalty
John Wright

So You Have Glaucoma | 1970 | $6·00
by E. R. Viers
Grune and Stratton 2nd edition

A Step by Step Guide to Personal Management for Blind Persons American Foundation for the Blind	1970	£2·25
You and Your Eyes *by* H. H. Prince A. H. and A. W. Reed (N.Z.)	1970	£1·25

FEET

Foot Care at all Ages by P. Read and H. Rosenstein British Medical Association Family Doctor Booklet	1964	15p
General Foot Care *by* P. H. Johnson John Wright	1969	50p
Trouble With Feet *by* M. Clarke Bell	1969	75p

FIRST AID

Accidents to Children: what to do in an emergency *by* M. Ellis Evans	1967	12s 6d o.p.
Baillière's Handbook of First Aid *revised by* S. Miles Baillière, Tindall 6th edition	1970	£1·00
First Aid Handbook *by* A. W. Gardener and P. I. Roylance Barker	1968	£1·05 o.p.
Modern First Aid *by* A. S. Playfair Hamlyn	1973	50p
New Safety and First Aid *by* A. W. Gardener and P. I. Roylance Pan Books	1970	30p

St. John Ambulance, St. Andrew's Ambulance Association and British Red Cross Society First Aid Manual St. John Ambulance Association 3rd edition	1972	40p

GENERAL

Avoidable Death: survival and commensense *by* J. Mansfield Cassell (on major killer diseases – bronchitis, heart disease, lung cancer, etc.)	1970	£1·80
Dictionary of Symptoms *by* J. Gomez Centaur	1967	£2·50
Paladin	1970	60p
Do Something About Your Health *by* M. Winstanley Tandem	1968	25p
Enjoy Life Longer: a guide to sixty of the leading spas *by* V. Graves and G. Graves Icon Books	1970	£2·25
Family Health Guide *edited by* S. Lock and A. Smith Reader's Digest	1972	£5·75
Home Medical Handbook *by* S. Charles Good Housekeeping Ebury Press	1973	£2·25
Home Truths for Home Doctors *by* M. Winstanley F. Muller	1963	90p o.p.
How Not To Die Young *by* J. Gomez G. Allen and Unwin	1973	£2·50

Know Your Illness *by* F. E. Graham-Bonnalie David and Charles	1973	£1·25
Structure and Function of the Body *by* C. P. Anthony Henry Kimpton 4th edition	1972	£2·25
The Will to Health *by* H. Williams Chest and Heart Association. Health Horizon Ltd.	1967	75p

HEADACHE

Do Something about that Migraine *by* K. M. Hay Tandem Books (available from Migraine Trust)	1968	20p
Migraine Office of Health Economics	1972	25p
Migraine *by* E. Hannington Priory Press Ltd.	1974	£2·50
Migraine: background and treatment *by* H. Maxwell J. Wright & Sons Ltd.	1966	75p
Migraine: the evolution of a common disorder *by* O. W. Sacks Faber and Faber	1970	£1·60
Relax *by* J. Madders BBC Publications	1973	65p
So Now You Know about Headaches *by* A. Elithorn British Medical Association Family Doctor Booklet	1971	15p

Treatment of Migraine *by* J. R. Graham J. and A. Churchill	1956	40p

HEARING

Conversations with the Deaf Royal National Institute for the Deaf		20p
The Deaf Child *by* E. Whetnall W. Heinemann	1971	£2·10
Deafness *by* J. Ballantyne J. and A. Churchill 2nd edition	1970	£2·25
Deafness – Let's Face It *by* T. H. Sutcliffe Royal National Institute for the Deaf (contains information on agencies that help hard of hearing)		25p
Hearing Aids Royal National Institute for the Deaf	1972	10p
Hearing Aids Which?	1973	
Hearing Aids, Lip Reading and Clear Speech *by* Sir A. and Lady C. Ewing Manchester University Press	1967	80p
Hearing and Not Hearing *by* H. Diack British Medical Association Family Doctor Booklet		15p
How Good Is Your Hearing? *by* E. Nendick Max Parish	1966	90p o.p.
How to Live with a Hearing Handicap *by* P. H. Van Itallie Faber and Faber	1965	£1·05

Journey into Loneliness *by* J. Ashley (autobiography) Bodley Head	1973	
Learning to Hear *by* E. Whetnall W. Heinemann	1970	£1·05
Plate Glass Prison *by* G. C. Firth Royal National Institute for the Deaf	1966	75p
Teaching Deaf Children to Talk *by* A. Ewing and C. Ewing Manchester University Press	1964	£1·80

HEART DISEASE

The Battle Against Heart Disease *by* P. E. Baldry Cambridge University Press	1971	£3·50
Coronary Case *by* R. Edwards (personal narrative) Faber and Faber	1964	50p
Do Something about those Arteries *by* H. T. N. Sears Tandem Books	1968	25p
Wingate-Baker	1969	£1·05
Don't Be Afraid of a Coronary *by* C. Watling Michael Joseph	1970	£1·50
Exercise and the Coronary Patient *by* E. R. Nye and P. Gay Wood Wolfe	1971	£1·00
Freedom from Heart Attacks *by* B. F. Miller and L. Galton Simon and Schuster (U.S.A.)	1972	$7·95

The Heart *by* D. Longmore World University Press Library Weidenfeld and Nicolson	1971	£2·00
Heart Attack: Are You a Candidate? *by* A. Blumenfield Erikson (New York)	1964	\$5·95
Heart Attack: you don't have to die *by* C. Barnard Allen	1972	£1·75
Heart Disease: some ways to prevent it *by* A. R. Southwood W. Heinemann	1962	17s 6d o.p.
Hearts *by* T. Thompson Michael Joseph (on the work of Dr Bakey and Cooley in the U.S.A.)	1972	£3·50
How Not to Get a Coronary *by* A. L. Wingfield British Medical Association Family Doctor Booklet		15p
How to Live with a Heart Attack *by* R. A. Miller Pelham Books	1973	£1·80
You Can Add Years to Your Heart *by* P. E. Norris Thorsons	1965	£1·00
Your Heart *by* H. Williams Cassell	1970	£1·80
Your Heart and How to Live with It *by* L. E. Lamb G. Allen and Unwin	1969	£2·25

HEIGHT

Human Growth After Birth *by* D. Sinclair Oxford University Press 2nd edition	1973	£2·00

HEREDITY

An ABC of Medical Genetics *by* C. O. Carter Lancet Publications	1969	75p
Genetics in Medicine *by* A. Smith Churchill Livingstone	1966	30p
Heredity in Humans *by* A. Scheinfeld Chatto and Windus	1972	£2·50
Human Genetics and Medicine *by* C. A. Clarke Edward Arnold	1970	£1·20 paperback 60p
The Porphyrias: study of inheritance and environment *by* G. Dean Pitman 2nd edition	1971	£3·25
Twins and Supertwins *by* A. Scheinfeld Penguin	1973	50p
Your Heredity and Environment *by* A. Scheinfeld Chatto and Windus	1973	£6·00

HORMONES

An ABC of Endocrinology *by* K. J. Catt Lancet Publications	1971	£1·00
Hormones: Chemical Communicators *by* R. Lewin Chapman	1972	75p

HOSPITALS

Children in Hospital *by* A. Hales-Tooke Priory Press Ltd.	1973	£2·50
Hospitals and Children: a parent's eye view *by* J. Robertson Gollancz	1962	90p o.p.
How to Survive in Hospital *by* K. Whitehorn Eyre Methuen	1972	85p
Know Your Hospital *by* L. Paine W. Heinemann Medical Books and British Hospital Journal	1972	65p
Let Us Tell You About Your Operation *by* G. Bunton British Medical Association Family Doctor Booklet	1974	15p
Play in Hospital *by* S. Harvey and A. Hales-Tooke Faber and Faber	1972	£3·00 & £1·40
So You Are Going into Hospital *by* T. Weston British Medical Association Family Doctor Booklet	1972	15p
Young Children in Hospitals *by* J. Robertson Tavistock Publications	1970	£1·00

YEARBOOKS

Handbook of the Association of Independent Hospitals and Kindred Organisations Association of Independent Hospitals	1974	75p
Hospitals and Health Services Yearbooks Institute of Health Administrators	1974	£9·85

HUNTINGTON'S CHOREA

Huntington's Chorea Committee on Huntingdon's Chorea of the Central Council for the Disabled and National Fund for Research into the Crippled Child Patients Booklet	1973	
National Fund for Research into Crippling Diseases (Available only through Patient's family doctor)		15p

ILEOSTOMY AND COLOSTOMY

All About a Colostomy *by* E. S. R. Hughes and E. M. Kyte Angus and Robertson	1969	£1·00
All About an Ileostomy *by* E. S. R. Hughes, E. M. Kyte and A. M. Cuthbertson Angus and Robertson	1972	£1·50
The Care of Your Colostomy *by* J. C. Goligher and M. Pollard Baillière, Tindall	1973	15p
The Care of your Ileostomy *by* J. C. Goligher and M. Pollard University of Leeds Department of Surgery, Leeds General Infirmary	1973	20p

IMMUNOLOGY

An ABC of Modern Immunology *by* E. S. Holborrow Lancet Publications	1973	75p

INFECTIOUS DISEASE

Common Colds and Related Diseases *by* D. A. Tyrell Edward Arnold	1965	£2·50

Communicable and Non Communicable Disease *by* K. L. Jones Canfield Press (San Francisco)	1970	£1·15
Dangerous People: where infection comes from and how to prevent it *by* E. Gundrey Spectator Publications	1967	£1·05
Fighting the Unseen: the story of viruses *by* S. Loebl Abelard-Schuman (U.S.A.)	1967	90p
Infectious Diseases: with chapters on venereal diseases *by* A. B. Christie Faber and Faber 5th edition	1968	£1·50
In Pursuit of the Common Cold *by* C. Andrewes W. Heinemann	1973	£3·35
The Natural History of Infectious Diseases *by* J. A. Boycott Edward Arnold	1971	£1·00 and 60p
Victory with Vaccines: the story of immunization *by* J. A. Parish Churchill Livingstone	1968	£1·50
Vitamin C and the Common Cold *by* L. Pauling Freeman (San Francisco)	1970	£1·90 and 80p
Ballantine Books	1972	30p

KIDNEY

The Human Kidney: what everyone should know *by* J. F. Mowbray and R. A. Parker Chest and Heart Association Health Horizon	1970	60p

MEN'S HEALTH

The Health of Men *by* R. J. Donaldson British Medical Association Family Doctor Booklet		15p
Your Prostrate *by* R. L. Rowan and P. Gillette Doubleday & Co. Inc.	1973	£2·70

MENTAL HEALTH

Anxiety, Nervousness and Depression *by* F. R. C. Casson British Medical Association Family Doctor Booklet		15p Corgi Mini Book 17½p
Clinical Psychiatry for the Layman *by* F. J. Fish J. Wright	1963	50p
Depression and its Treatment *by* J. Pollitt W. Heinemann Medical Books Ltd.	1965	£1·20
Depression, the blue plague *by* C. A. H. Watts Priory Press Ltd.	1965	£1·20
Emotional Problems *by* P. Fletcher Pan Books	1972	40p
Exploring the Mind: man's search for mental health *by* S. Loebl Abelhard-Schuman (U.S.A.)		£1·50
Fears and Phobias *by* I. M. Marks W. Heinemann Medical Books Ltd.	1969	£2·50

Insight: a guide to psychiatry and psychiatric services *by* B. Kenny and T. Whitehead Croom Helm	1973	£4·00 and £1·95
The Mending of Minds: psychiatric illness and its treatment, a guide for families and patients *by* W. L. Tonge Darwen, Finlayson	1970	£1·75
Mind and Body *by* S. Black Kimber	1969	£3·15
Peace from Nervous Suffering *by* C. Weekes Angus and Robertson	1972	£1·50
Phobias: their nature and control *by* S. Rachman Thomas (Springfield, U.S.A.)	1968	$5·75
Self Help for your Nerves *by* C. Weekes Angus and Robertson	(1969) 1973	£1·60
Understanding Anxiety in Every Day Life *by* E. Trimmer G. Allen and Unwin	1970	£1·25
Understanding Your Nerves *by* J. A. Parr David and Charles	1971	£2·50
Your Doctor's Guide to Living with Stress *by* F. Graham-Bonnalie David and Charles	1972	£1·95

PSYCHOLOGY AND PSYCHOTHERAPY

All About the Human Mind *by* R. M. Golbenson W. H. Allen	1965	£1·25
Healing the Sick Mind *by* H. Guntrip G. Allen and Unwin	1964	£1·05 and 50p

I'm O.K. – You're O.K.: a practical guide to transactional analysis *by* T. A. Harris Cape	1973	£2·25
An Introduction to Psychotherapy: its history and modern schools of thought *by* J. A. Hadfield G. Allen and Unwin	1967	£3·00
Know Your Own Mind *by* H. J. Walton British Medical Association Family Doctor Booklet	1973	15p
The Patient and the Analyst *by* J. Sander et al G. Allen and Unwin	1973	£2·95
Psychotherapy: do we need more talking treatment? National Association for Mental Health. Mind Report No. 12 NAMH Bookstall Services	1974	20p
Try Being Human *by* A. Forbes Langdon Books	1973	£1·80

Transcendental Meditation

Tranquillity Without Pills *by* J. Robbins and D. Fisher Souvenir Press	1972	£2·00 o.p.

MENTAL HEALTH SERVICES

A History of the Mental Health Services *by* K. Jones Routledge	1972	£5·00
Mental Illness in the Family: advice for relations on some practical problems National Association for Mental Health	1972	7½p

Mental Subnormality | 1967 | 50p
by W. A. Heaton-Ward
J. Wright 3rd edition
(covers 1959 Mental Health Act – guide for magistrates, mental welfare officers, social workers, etc.)

NAMH Guide to the Mental Health Act 1959 | | 30p
by A. Hargrove
National Association for Mental Health

Patients' Rights: the mentally disordered in hospital | 1973 | 20p
National Association for Mental Health. Mind Report No. 10
(available from the NAMH Bookshop)

Psychiatric Emergencies and the Law | 1968 | £1·70
by P. E. Kenyon
J. Wright

Treatment and Care in Mental Illness | 1971 | 85p
Consumers Association

MULTIPLE SCLEROSIS AND PARAPLEGIA

Dramatic Revival | 1972 (August)
by R. MacDougall (author's recovery from M.S. through gluten free diet)
Daily Telegraph Magazine

Living at Your Best with Multiple Sclerosis: a handbook for patients | 1972 | $7·95 and $4·95
by G. H. Hess
Thomas (Springfield, U.S.A.)

Multiple Sclerosis | 1971 | £3·38
by J. H. D. Millar
Thomas (Springfield, U.S.A.)

Multiple Sclerosis: a Reappraisal | 1972 | £6·00
by D. MacAlpine et al.
Churchill Livingstone

Multiple Sclerosis and Me *by* M. H. Greenblatt Thomas (Springfield, U.S.A.)	1972	£2·45
Still at Home with Multiple Sclerosis Multiple Sclerosis Society (replaces At Home with Multiple Sclerosis)	1972	30p

MYASTHENIA GRAVIS

Living with Myasthenia Gravis *by* J. W. Kempton Thomas (Springfield, U.S.A.)	1972	$6·95

PARAPLEGIA

Bring Me My Bow *by* M. Harriman (autobiography) Gollancz	1967	£1·75 o.p.
Horizontal Man *by* M. Harriman (autobiography) Longmans	1964	80p o.p.
Polio is not for Pity *by* I. Holdsworth (autobiography) G. Allen and Unwin	1963	£1·00 o.p.
The Polio Story *by* P. J. Fisher W. Heinemann Medical Books	1967	£1·75
Understanding Paraplegia *by* J. J. Walsh Tavistock Publications	1964	£1·05
What Price Polio? *by* P. Walton (autobiography) Allen and Wingate	1959	12s 6d o.p.

PARKINSON'S DISEASE

Parkinson's Disease: a booklet for patients and their families *by* R. B. Godwin-Austen Parkinson's Disease Society of the United Kingdom	1972	

NATIONAL HEALTH SERVICE

Complaints against Doctors: a study in professional accountability *by* R. Klein Knight	1973	£4·00
The Doctor and the Law *by* J. Leary Taylor Pitman Medical and Scientific Publishing Co. Ltd. (written for medical profession)	1970	£2·00
Doctors and State Medicine *by* G. Forsyth Pitman Medical Publishing Co. 2nd edition	1973	£2·00
Family Guide to the Law Reader's Digest	1971	£5·50
Law of Doctor and Patient *by* S. R. Speller H. K. Lewis (written for medical profession)	1973	£5·00
National Health Service and You News of the World	1970	o.p.
Patients, Practitioners and Medical Care: aspects of medical sociology *by* D. Robinson W. Heinemann	1973	£1·15
Some Lesser-known Services and Concessions Available under the National Health Service Patients' Association	1973	Gratis

NOISE

The Law on Noise Noise Abatement Society	1969	£1·05
Noise *by* R. Taylor Penguin	1970	35p

Noise and Man *by* W. Burns J. Murray 2nd edition	1973	£5·00

NUTRITION

Coeliac Handbook Coeliac Society H. K. Lewis and Foyle's Medical Department	1971	80p
Cooking for the Sick and Convalescent *by* N. Heaton and V. H. Mottram Faber and Faber		£1·37½
Diet Without Tears Cookerybook *by* I. H. Rogers H. K. Lewis 3rd edition (for diabetics)	1973	65p
Diets for Sick Children *by* D. M. Francis Blackwell	1974	£4·00
Enjoying Your Restricted Diet *by* M. B. Salmon and A. Quigley Thomas (Springfield, U.S.A.)	1973	$10·75
Food Facts and Fallacies *by* A. C. Cameron Faber and Faber	1973	80p
Food Values of Portions Commonly Used *by* A. Bowes and C. Church Lippincott (Philadelphia, U.S.A.)	1970	£2·70
Healthy Eating for the Elderly Healthy Eating in Pregnancy British Nutrition Foundation Pamphlets		8p each inc. postage
Human Nutrition *by* V. H. Mottram Edward Arnold 2nd edition	1972	£1·75

The Low Fat Cholesterol Diet *by* C. B. Y. Bond et al Doubleday (N.Y.)	1971	£3·75
Low Salt Diets *by* M. Toohey and R. Taylor British Medical Association Family Doctor Booklet		15p
Manual of Nutrition Ministry of Agriculture, Fisheries and Food H.M.S.O. 7th edition	1970	47p
Measure for Measure Cookery Book *by* Elizabeth O'Reilly Heinemann Health Books (for diabetics and weightwatchers)	1974	£2·10
Nutrition and Dietetic Foods *by* A. E. Bender Leonard Hill Books	1973	£3·50
Nutrition and its Disorders *by* P. S. McClaren Churchill Livingstone	1972	£1·50
Second Book of Food and Nutrition *by* W. Matthews and D. Wells Home Economics in Association with the Flour Advisory Bureau	1973	£1·80
Soothing Food: a new view of cooking for ulcers and difficult stomachs *by* B. Duncan Faber and Faber	1972	£2·25
So You Need a Diet *by* R. Kemp British Medical Association Family Doctor Booklet	1969	15p
The Good, the Bad and the Fattening: a dictionary of food *by* D. Wells Times Books	1975	£3·25

The Value of Food 1970 80p
by P. Fisher and A. Bender
Oxford University Press

SLIMMING

Anorexia Nervosa 1969 £1·50
by P. Dally
W. Heinemann

Complete Slimmer 1964 £1·50
by J. Yudkin o.p.
MacGibbon and Kee

Doctors' Quick Weight Loss Diet 1970 25p
by I. M. Stillman and S. S. Baker
Pan

Eat Fat and Grow Slim 1968
by R. Mackarness o.p.
Harvill

Eating Disorders: obesity, anorexia nervosa and the person within 1973 £3·95
by H. Bruch
Routledge and Kegan Paul

Lose Weight and Live Normally without Diet and Exercise 1973 £3·00
by A. Fewster
Pelham Books

Obesity and its Management 1973 £2·50
by D. Craddock
Churchill Livingstone 2nd edition

Overweight: causes, cost and control 1968 £3·55
by J. Mayer
Prentice-Hall (N. Jersey, U.S.A.)
Spectrum Books £1·25

Overweight: slimming made easy 1973 £1·95
by J. A. Parr
Arthur Baker Ltd.

Sustained Weight Control: the individual approach | 1973 | £1·00

by T. S. Danowski
Blackwell 2nd edition

This Slimming Business | 1970 | 30p

by J. Yudkin
Penguin

The Truth about Weight Control: how to lose weight permanently | 1973 | £2·50

by N. Solomon and S. Sheppard
G. Allen and Unwin

OCCUPATIONAL HEALTH

Effects of Abnormal Physical Conditions at Work | 1967 | £1·05

edited by C. N. Davies et al
British Occupational Hygiene Society et al. Conference Report
E. and S. Livingstone

Employment Medical Advisory Service Act 1972: a guide to the service | 1973 | Gratis

Department of Employment
H.M.S.O.

First Aid in the Factory | 1973 | £1·20

by Lord Taylor et al
Longman Group 4th edition

A Guide to Industrial Safety and Health | 1968 | £1·80

edited by R. Packman
Longmans

Hazards of Work: how to fight them | 1973 | £2·70 hardback and 90p

by P. Kinnersly
Pluto Press 1973

Hearing and Noise in Industry | 1970 | £1·75

by W. Burns and D. W. Robinson
H.M.S.O.

Industrial Dermatitis: precautionary measures 1969 12½p
H.M. Factory Inspectorate Safety Health and Welfare Booklets. N.S. No. 18 o.p.
Department of Employment and Productivity
H.M.S.O.

Industrial Dermatoses and the Industrial Injuries Act 1968 50p
by J. T. Ingram
Churchill Livingstone

Safety Uncensored 1971 35p
by J. Tye and K. Lillyett
London Transworld (Corgi Books)

The Way Back: the patient with work problems Gratis
Department of Employment pamphlets on rehabilitation for the blind, special help for severely disabled, industrial rehabilitation units
(Available from any Employment Exchange or Department of Employment Administrative Headquarters)

PREGNANCY

Advice to the Expectant Mother 1973 30p
by J. J. Browne
edited by J. C. M. Browne
Churchill Livingstone 14th edition

At Your Best for Birth and Later 1969 40p
by E. Montgomery
John Wright 3rd edition

Before Birth: fact and fallacy 1965 90p
by E. Trimmer o.p.
MacGibbon and Kee

Breast Feeding 1968 20p
by F. P. Roberts
John Wright

A Child is Born 1965 £1·50
by P. Dally and R. Sweering
P. Owen

Dictionary of Pregnancy: childbirth and contraception *by* H. A. Brant and M. Brant Mayflower	1971	80p and 35p
Enlightened Childbirth *by* E. E. Joslin J. Wright	1965	40p
First Nine Months of Life *by* G. L. Flanagan W. Heinemann Medical Books Ltd.	1970	90p
Have Your Baby – Keep Your Figure *by* M. B. Davies and E. Maisel Arlington Books	1964	75p
Budget books		60p
Sphere		25p
Having a Baby *by* J. F. Robinson Churchill Livingstone	1965	50p
The Know-how of Breast Feeding *by* S. Close J. Wright	1972	40p
The Know-how of Infant Care *by* S. Close J. Wright 2nd edition	1972	40p
The Know-how of Infant Feeding *by* S. Close J. Wright 3rd edition	1973	40p
The Know-how of Pregnancy and Labour *by* S. Close J. Wright	1969	50p
Preparing for Childbirth: a manual for expectant parents *by* F. W. Goodrich G. Allen and Unwin	1967	£1·50

Your Baby and Your Figure: ante and postnatal exercises — 1972 — 15p
by L. P. Burns
E. and S. Livingstone 3rd edition

NATURAL CHILDBIRTH

Dick Read's Childbirth Without Fear: the principles and practice of natural childbirth — 1968 — £1·00
edited by L. Snaith and A. Coxon
W. Heinemann Medical Books Ltd. 5th edition

Sex Development and Maternity: childbirth without pain by the psychoprophylactic method — 1968 — £2·50
by P. Vellay
Hutchinson; now G. Allen and Unwin

A Way to Natural Childbirth — 1973 — 75p
by H. Heardman
revised by M. Ebner
Churchill Livingstone

CONTRACEPTION

Conception, Birth and Contraception — 1969 — £1·05
by R. J. Demarest and J. J. Sciarra
Hodder and Stoughton

Contraception Today: report of a conference held in 1970 — 1971 — £1·00
Family Planning Association

Contraceptives 'Which?' — 1972 — £1·00
Consumers Association

Dictionary of Pregnancy: childbirth and contraception — 1971 — 80p
35p
by H. A. Brant and M. Brant
Mayflower

Family Planning — 1969 — 15p
by M. Smith
British Medical Association Family Doctor Booklet
Corgi Minibooks — 1971 — 17½p

Family Planning *by* J. F. Robinson Churchill Livingstone	1967	25p
Intrauterine Devices *by* C. Wood Butterworth	1971	£1·00
Male Methods of Birth Control *by* G. R. Scott Luxor Press	1971	30p
Motherhood and the Safe Time Simplified *by* J. L. Cameron Churchill Livingstone	1964	5p
Planning for a Family: an atlas of temperature charts *by* J. Marshall Faber and Faber	1969 (1965)	50p paperback
Vasectomy and Vasectomania *by* D. and H. Wolfers Mayflower	1974	50p

REPRODUCTION

From Conception to Birth *by* R. Rugh and L. B. Shettles G. Allen and Unwin	1972	£6·00
From Sterility to Fertility: a guide to causes and cure of childlessness *by* E. Philipp Thorsons	1957	o.p.
Impotence and Frigidity *by* D. W. Hastings Churchill Livingstone	1963	£3·00
Infertility Consumers Association	1972	75p
Reproduction and Environment *by* R. Holmes Oliver and Boyd	1968	37½p

Sex: an account of its functions and effects in reproduction *by* S. Michelmore Eyre and Spottiswode	1964	£1·05 o.p.
Utopian Motherhood: new trends in human reproduction *by* R. T. Francoeur G. Allen and Unwin	1970	£2·75

RHEUMATISM AND ARTHRITIS

Aches, Pains and Rheumatism: a sufferer's guide *by* A. St. J. Dixon British Medical Association Family Doctor Booklet	1973	15p
All Out Against Arthritis *by* F. C. Lewis Prentice-Hall (U.S.A.)	1973	$5·95
Answer to Arthritis *by* C. Peterson F. Fell Inc. (N.Y., U.S.A.)	1968	£1·15
Arthritis and Back Pain *by* J. C. Adams Medical and Technical Publishing Co. Ltd	1972	£2·50
Arthritis and Rheumatism *by* W. S. Copeman Evans Brothers Ltd.	1967	75p o.p.
The Arthritis Handbook: a patient's manual on rheumatism and arthritis and gout *by* D. C. Crain Arlington Books	1971	$6·50 and £1·45 Arco
Arthritis: help in your own hands *by* H. B. MacFarlane Thorsons	1970	30p

Beyond the Copper Bracelet: what you should know about arthritis *by* L. A. Healey and K. R. Wilske Thomas (Springfield, U.S.A.)	1972	£1·48
Do Something about that Rheumatism *by* J. L. Struthers Tandem	1969	25p
Wingate-Baker		£1·05
Home Care of Arthritis *by* R. C. Lewis Blackwell (Lippincott, U.S.A.)	1971	50p
Marriage, Sex and Arthritis Arthritis and Rheumatism Council	1973	10p
Understanding Rheumatism *by* T. R. Littler Tavistock Publications	1966	£1·25

SCHIZOPHRENIA

How to Live with Schizophrenia *by* A. Hoffer and H. Osmand Johnson	1966	£1·50
Living with Schizophrenia National Schizophrenia Fellowship	1974	62p
Marriage and Fertility of Women Suffering from Schizophrenia or Affective Disorders *by* B. C. Stevens Oxford University Press	1969	£3·00
Sanity, Madness and the Family: families of schizophrenics *by* R. D. Laing and E. Esterson Tavistock Publications	1970	£2·75
Penguin		40p
Schizophrenia *by* A. R. K. Mitchell Priory Press Ltd.	1972	80p

Schizophrenia: the divided mind *by* J. Emerson and C. Wallace British Medical Association Family Doctor Booklet	1969	15p
Soul Murder: persecution in the family *by* M. Schatzman Allen Lane	1973	£2·50
This Stranger My Son: a mother's story *by* L. Wilson John Murray	1968	£1·50

SEX

A Doctor Speaks on Sexual Expression in Marriage *by* D. W. Hastings Churchill Livingstone 2nd edition	1971	£3·50
Facts of Sex *by* J. James MacGibbon and Kee	1969	90p
Panther		30p
Fundamentals of Sex *by* P. Cauthery and M. Cole W. H. Allen	1971	£3·00
Corgi Books	1973	50p
Males and Females *by* C. Hutt Penguin	1972	60p
Man and Woman: the basis of their relationship *by* K. H. Wrage Collins	1969	£3·50
Modern Marriage *by* E. F. Griffeth Methuen	1973	£1·10
People in Love: a modern guide to sex in marriage *by* C. Rayner Hamlyn	1968	62½p

Sex and Gender: on the development of masculinity and femininity *by* R. J. Stoller Hogarth Press	1968	£3·00
Sex and Love *by* J. Hemming and Z. Maxwell W. Heinemann Educational Books	(1972) 1973	£1·50
Sex and the Longer Life *by* I. Felstein Penguin	1970	£1·25
Sex and the Married Woman *by* E. Chesser Corgi Books	1970	35p
Sex in the Middle Years *by* W. Greengross National Marriage Guidance Council	1969	25p
Sex: the plain facts *by* J. Bevan Faber and Faber	(1966) 1969	90p and 45p
Sexual Life After Sixty *by* S. Rubin G. Allen and Unwin	1966	£2·00
Sexual Myths and Fallacies *by* J. L. McCary Van Nostrand, Reinhold	1972	£3·50
Sexuality and Subnormality *edited by* G. Katz National Society for Mentally Handicapped Children	1972	50p
So Now You Know About Sex *by* E. Penrose British Medical Association Family Doctor Booklet	1972	15p
Understanding Sex: a young person's guide *by* A. F. Guttmacher G. Allen and Unwin	1971	£1·95

Sex Education

Boy into Man: sex knowledge for the growing boy *by* D. and A. Hilton Denholm House Press	1972	15p
Facts of Life *by* C. Greet Stacey	1972	35p
Girl into Woman: sex knowledge for the growing girl *by* D. and A. Hilton Denholm House Press (aimed at 11–13 years)	1972	15p
How Human Life Begins *by* J. J. Head Murray	1970	£1·50 and £1·05
How You Began *by* H. Spiers Dent (aimed at 4–8 years)	1971	75p and 45p
How Your Life Began *by* R. Pilkington British Medical Association Family Doctor Booklet	1972	15p
Sex Education *by* M. Hill and M. Lloyd-Jones National Secular Society	1970	25p
Sex Education: learning to live with sex Family Planning Association (aimed at teenagers)	1972	25p
Sex in a Young Man's Life *by* E. K. Morris National Christian Education Council	1971	55p

Sexual Deviations

Homosexuality *by* F. Kenyon British Medical Association Family Doctor Booklet	1973	15p
Homosexuality *by* D. J. West Penguin	1969	35p
Duckworth revised edition	1968	£2·10
Homosexuality: its nature, causation and treatment *by* C. Allen Staples	1958	75p
Homosexuality: some questions and answers Albany Trust	1969	15p
Human Aspects of Sexual Deviations *by* E. Chesser Jarrolds	1971	£2·25
Arrow Books		40p
Love Between Women *by* C. Wolffe Duckworth	1971	£2·50
Odd Men Out: homosexuality in men and women *by* E. Chesser Gollancz	1959	12s 6d o.p.
Sexual Variations *by* J. Randell Priory Press Ltd.	1973	£2·50

SKIN

Management of Common Skin Diseases *by* C. P. A. Dupont Henry Kimpton	1973	£1·25
Your Skin and the Body Beautiful *by* P. J. Hare British Medical Association Family Doctor Booklet		15p

SLEEP DISORDERS

About Sleep *by* A. H. Duncan Thorsons	1964	30p
Children and Sleep *by* R. S. Illingworth Family Health Publications	1958	o.p.
Conquer Insomnia *by* M. N. Pai Souvenir and Arlington Books	1965	25p
Insomnia: the guide for troubled sleepers *by* G. C. Luce and J. Segal Longmans	1970	£2·50
Sleep *by* I. Oswald Penguin	1966	30p
Sleep Disorders: searchlight on *by* M. N. Pai Lit. Services	1969	£1·80 and 75p
So Now You Know About Sleeping and Not Sleeping *by* I. Oswald British Medical Association Family Doctor Booklet	1970	15p

SLEEP LEARNING

Learning and Sleep: the theory and practice of hypnopaedia *by* F. Rubin J. Wright	1971	£1·75

SOCIAL SERVICES

Administrative Tribunals *by* R. E. Wraith and P. G. Hutchinson Royal Institute of Public Administration G. Allen and Unwin		£5·75

Accidents and the Law Law Society and Oyez Publishing	1974	
Battered Women: Interaction advisory service Chiswick Women's Aid	1973	
Before You See a Solicitor *by* G. Sanctuary Law Society and Oyez Publishing		60p
Chiswick Women's Aid Aims and Objectives Inter-Action Advisory Service for Chiswick Women's Aid	1973	
Claimant of Client: a social worker's view of the supplementary benefits commission *by* O. Stevenson G. Allen and Unwin	1973	£4·25
Common Human Needs *by* C. Towle *edited by* E. Younghusband G. Allen and Unwin	1973	£3·15
Consumer's Guide to the British Social Services *by* P. Willmott Penguin 3rd edition	1973	50p
Half way Houses: Richmond Fellowship brochure and leaflets on sheltered accommodation run by the fellowship for alcoholics, schizophrenics, ex drug addicts, adolescents, and families and people needing minimal support		20p
Home Help Service in England and Wales Government Social Survey H.M.S.O.	1972	£2·00
Public Social Services: handbook of information *edited by* P. Willmott Bedford Square Press of National Council of Social Service	1973	£1·25

Rogues and Vagabonds: a survey of legislation relevant to the long term homeless *by* R. Smith No Fixed Abode	1973	10p
Single Mothers: survival notes Mothers in Action	1973	15p
Social Isolation of the Single Woman and her Dependants National Council for Single Women and her Dependants	1973	10p
Tribunals and Inquiries: a guide to procedure *by* N. Van Dyke Oyez Publishing	1965	£3·00
Unsupported Mothers and the Care of their Children Mothers in Action	1970	25p
Welfare State: its aims, benefits and costs *by* J. F. Sleeman G. Allen and Unwin	1973	£3·85
Women's Rights: a practical guide *by* A. Coote and T. Gill Penguin Special	1973	60p

SPEECH

Aphasia and Other Aspects of Language *by* M. Critchley Edward Arnold	1970	£9·75
Aphasia Handbook for Adults and Children *by* A. Agranowitz and M. R. McKeown Thomas (Springfield, U.S.A.)	1964	
Child with Delayed Speech *by* M. Rutter and J. A. M. Martin W. Heinemann	1972	£3·50
Developmental Aphasia: an introduction *by* P. Griffiths Invalid Children's Aid Association	1972	30p

Dysphasia: professional guidance for family and patient *by* M. Buck Prentice-Hall (N. Jersey, U.S.A.)	1968	£3·50
A History of the Treatment of Speech Disorders *by* M. Eldridge Livingstone	1968	£1.50
An Introduction to Stuttering *by* F. B. Robinson Prentice Hall (New Jersey, U.S.A.)	1964	£3·65
Singer's and Actor's Throat: vocal mechanism of the professional user and its care in health and disease *by* N. A. Punt W. Heinemann 2nd edition	1967	90p
Speech and Reason *by* W. Abse John Wright (U. Press of Virginia)	1971	£5·50
Speech Delay: its treatment by speech play: a book for parents *by* M. Craft John Wright	1969	75p
Speech Disorders in Children *by* C. E. Renfrew Pergamon	1972	£1·25
The Voice and its Disorders *by* M. C. L. Greene Pitman Medical Publishing Ltd.	1972	£2·25
Voice Articulation *by* C. Van Riper and J. V. Irwin Pitman Medical Publishing Co.	1959	£2·75
Why Stammer? *by* H. St. John Rumsey Faber	1957	o.p.

STROKES

All About Strokes *by* A. B. Carter Nelson	1968	£2·10

Coping with a Stroke Illness *by* H. Williams Chest and Heart Association	1971	10p
Help Yourselves: a handbook for hemiplegics and their families *by* P. E. Jay et al Butterworth 2nd edition	1972	75p
Helping the Stroke Patient to Speak *by* W. Kingdom-Ward Churchill Livingstone	1969	£1·25
Return to Independence: exercises for stroke patients *by* T. Wareham Chest and Heart Association	1970	40p
A Stroke in the Family *by* V. E. Griffith Penguin	1970	25p
Stroke: a diary of recovery *by* D. Ritchie (autobiography) Faber and Faber	1974	£1·10
Strokes and How to Live with Them *by* A. B. Carter British Medical Association Family Doctor Booklet		15p
The Third Killer: meditations on a stroke *by* G. Wint (autobiography) Chatto and Windus	1965	£1·50 o.p.

SURGERY

A Change of Face and Figure *by* I. Felstein Constable	1971	£2·10
Let Us Tell You About Your Operation *by* G. Bunton British Medical Association Family Doctor Booklet	1974	15p

Tonsils and Adenoids 15p
by D. N. F. Harrison
British Medical Association Family Doctor Booklet

TERMINAL CARE

Care of the Dying 1973 £2·50
by R. Lammerton
Priory Press Ltd.

Care of the Dying: a report of a symposium held 29th November, 1972 1973 65p
Department of Health and Social Security.
Reports on Health and Social Subjects No. 5
H.M.S.O.

Life Before Death 1973 £5·95
by A. Cartwright, L. Hockey and J. L. Anderson
Routledge and Kegan Paul

The Puzzle of Pain 1973 75p
by R. Melzack

TRANSPLANTATION

A Gift of Life: observations on organ transplantation 1970 £2·25
by R. Calne
Medical and Technical Publishing Co.

Law on Human Transplants and Bequests of Bodies 1970 £3·00 and £4·50
by W. A. J. Farndale
White's Publishers. Ravenwood Publications

Organ Transplants: the moral issues 1970 90p
by C. Lyons
S.C.M. Press
Penguin

A Second Look at Life: transplantation and dialyisis patients: their own stories 1973
edited by F. T. Rapaport
Grune and Stratton N.Y. and London

Spare Part Surgery: the surgical practice of the future *by* D. Longmore Aldus Books	1968	£1·12½ and 80p

UNORTHODOX MEDICINE

Fringe Medicine *by* B. Inglis Faber and Faber	1964	£1·90

ACUPUNCTURE

Acupuncture *by* M. Duke Constable	1973	£2·50 and £1·25
Acupuncture *by* F. Mann W. Heinemann 2nd edition	1971	£3·10
Acupuncture and You *by* L. Moss Citadel Press 2nd edition	1972	£2·00
The Healing Needles *by* C. Ewart Elm Tree Books. Hamish Hamilton	1972	£1·70
A Layman's Guide to Acupuncture *by* Y. Manaka and I. Urquart Phaidon Press	1972	£2·75

CHIROPRACTICE

Chiropractice *by* A. G. Scofield Thorsons	1968	£2·50

HOMOEOPATHY

Essentials of Homoeopathic prescribing *by* H. F. Woods Health and Science Press	1970	75p
An Introduction to the Principle and Practice of Homoeopathy *by* C. E. Wheeler Health Science Press 3rd edition	1971	£2·75

The Principles and Art of Cure by Homoeopathy *by* A. H. Roberts Health Science Press 2nd edition	1972	£2·00

RADIESTHESIA

Health, radiation and Healing *by* M. Ash Darton, Longman and Todd	1962	90p o.p.
An Introduction to Medical Radiesthesia and radionics *by* V. Wethered C. W. Daniel & Co. Ltd.	1974	£2·75
Matter in the Making *by* L. Day and G. De La Warr Vincent and Stuart	1966	£1·80

VARICOSE VEINS

On the Causation of Varicose Veins: their prevention and arrest by natural means *by* L. Cleave John Wright	1960	40p
Varicose Veins *by* R. Foote John Wright	1960	£3·60

VENEREAL DISEASE

Infectious Diseases: with chapters on venereal diseases *by* A. B. Christie Faber and Faber 5th edition	1968	£2·50
Microbes and Morals: the strange story of venereal disease *by* T. Rosebury Viking Press (N.Y.) Secker and Warburg	1971 1972	£3·10
Sexually Transmitted Diseases *by* P. Silver Churchill Livingstone	1972	£1·25

V.D. and Diseases Transmitted Sexually *by* R. S. Morton British Medical Association Family Doctor Booklet	1968	15p
Corgi Minibooks	1971	17½p
V.D. Explained *by* R. Statham Priory Press Ltd.	1972	£2·25 and 80p

WOMEN'S HEALTH

Change of Life *by* M. Landau British Medical Association Family Doctor Booklet		15p
The Change of Life *by* W. Richards L. J. Speight	1974	£3·50
Everywoman: a gynaecological guide for life *by* D. Llewllyn-Jones Faber and Faber	1971	£2·25 60p
Femina: a manual of sex hygiene *by* E. Trimmer MacGibbon and Kee	1966	£1·25
Mayflower	1968	25p
Feminine Forever *by* R. A. Wilson W. H. Allen	1968	90p
Health of Women British Medical Association Family Doctor Booklet	1974	
The Menstrual Cycle *by* K. Dalton W. Heinemann	1969	25p Penguin
The Middle Years: the change of life *by* A. Sharman E. and S. Livingstone	1962	50p

Our Bodies, Ourselves *by* the Boston Women's Health Collective	1972	
On Being a Woman: the book that removes fear *by* W Gifford-Jones W. Heinemann Medical	1971	90p
Pre-menstrual Syndrome *by* K. Dalton W. Heinemann	1964	£1·20
Principles and Practice of Hormone Therapy in Gynaecology and Obstetrics *by* J. Uffer W. de Gruyter (Berlin)	1969	
Understanding Cystitis *by* A. Kilmartin W. Heinemann Health Books	1973	£1·00
Woman: the middle years *by* M. Smith British Medical Association Family Doctor Booklet	1970	15p
Women of Forty: a menopausal syndrome *by* M. E. Landau Faber and Faber 2nd edition	1964	70p

REFERENCE WORKS

Black's Medical Dictionary *edited by* W. A. Thomson A. and C. Black 29th edition	1971	£2·75
Charities Digest Family Welfare Association 81st edition	1974	£2·00
Dictionary of Abbreviations in Medicine and the Related Sciences *by* E. Steen Cassell 3rd edition	1971	£1·25

Directory of Voluntary Organisations Concerned with Children *edited by* M. L. K. Pringle et al Longmans for National Bureau of Co-operation in Child Care	1969	£3·50
Handbook of the Association of Independent Hospitals and Kindred Organisations Association of Independent Hospitals	1974	75p
Handbook of Organisations Relating to the Health and Social Services Health and Social Services Journal. Kings Fund Centre	1973	20p
Hospitals and Health Services Yearbook Institute of Health Service Administrators	1974	£9·95
Medical Directory Churchill Livingstone 2v. annual	1973 1974	
Medical Register General Medical Council 2v. annual	1973 1974	
Pears Medical Encyclopaedia *edited by* J. A. C. Brown Pelham new edition	1971	£3·50
Social Services in Britain Central Office of Information H.M.S.O. 91st edition	1973	75p
Some Nursing Homes (England and Wales) Chest and Heart Association (lists 400 residences catering for invalids)	1970	40p
Stedman's Medical Directory Churchill Livingstone 22nd edition	1972	£8·00

Index